STANDARDS, JOB DESCRIPTIONS, AND PERFORMANCE EVALUATIONS FOR NURSING PRACTICE

STANDARDS, JOB DESCRIPTIONS, AND PERFORMANCE EVALUATIONS FOR NURSING PRACTICE

Dale Kayser Jernigan, R.N., M.S.N.
Director of Nursing Service
South Baldwin Hospital
Foley, Alabama

Abigail Pepper Young, R.N., B.S.N.
Director of Inservice Education
South Baldwin Hospital
Foley, Alabama

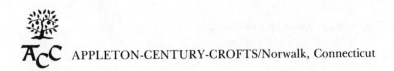 APPLETON-CENTURY-CROFTS/Norwalk, Connecticut

0-8385-8673-2

Prentice-Hall International, Inc., London
Prentice-Hall of Australia, Pty. Ltd., Sydney
Prentice-Hall Canada, Inc.
Prentice-Hall of India Private Limited, New Delhi
Prentice-Hall of Japan, Inc., Tokyo
Prentice-Hall of Southeast Asia (Pte.) Ltd., Singapore
Whitehall Books Ltd., Wellington, New Zealand
Editora Prentice-Hall do Brasil Ltda., Rio de Janeiro

Library of Congress Cataloging in Publication Data

Jernigan, Dale Kayser.
   Standards, job descriptions, and performance evaluation for nursing practice.

   Bibliography: p.
   Includes index.
   1. Nursing—Standards. 2. Nurses—Job descriptions. 3. Nursing—Rating of. 4. Nursing—Standards—United States. 5. Nurses—United States—Job descriptions. 6. Nurses—United States—Rating of. I. Young, Abigail Pepper. II. Title. [DNLM: 1. Nursing care—Standards. 2. Nursing service, Hospital—Organization and administration. WY 105 J55s]
   RT85.5.J47   1983   610.73′068′3   82-24482
   ISBN 0-8385-8673-2

Cover and text design: Lynn M. Luchetti

PRINTED IN THE UNITED STATES OF AMERICA

To the Nurses of South Baldwin Hospital

Contents

Preface

Well-defined job descriptions have always been necessary to nursing practice. In recent years, however, concepts involving "standards" and "quality assurance" have promoted changes in the focus of nursing practice from simply job descriptions to integrated systems. Nurse professionals are challenged to set high standards of practice, and to develop and implement techniques to achieve these standards. In response to this challenge, the material in this book was developed.

The purpose of this book is to integrate the nursing process into standards of practice, job descriptions, and performance evaluations, utilizing systems theory. The main emphasis will be not only the interrelationship of these standards, job descriptions, and performance evaluations, but also their relation to the delivery of patient care.

Nursing service administrators will find this book very useful in meeting the Joint Commission on Accreditation of Hospital's Nursing Service Standards. Specifically, Standard II in the Accreditation Manual states:

> The nursing department/service shall be organized to meet the nursing care needs of patients and to maintain established standards of nursing practice.

Further, this Standard requires the establishment of standards of nursing care and criteria-based performance evaluations that reflect the job descriptions. Measures must be taken to evaluate the nursing care provided, as described in the standards of nursing care.[1]

When our 82-bed general hospital was surveyed by the Joint Commission in June of 1981, the nurse surveyor not only approved this material, but also praised and recommended it to other hospitals. The key factor differentiating this material from other work was the integrated standards of practice, job descriptions, and performance evaluations based upon the nursing process. From the numerous calls and requests we received for copies of this material, we determined that there was a need to have it published.

The American Nurses' Association is credited as the main source for the writing of the standards of nursing practice presented in this book. Our standards were derived directly from the ANA's Standards for Maternal-Child Health Nursing Practice,[2] Cardiovascular Nursing Practice,[3] Standards of Nursing Practice: Operating Room,[4] Medical-Surgical Nursing Practice,[5] and Emergency Nursing Practice.[6] These standards were reorganized into the four phases relating to the nursing process, and revised to meet the needs of our nursing service.

There are many types and varieties of nursing standards of practice. Our intent is not to present our standards for universal use, but to demonstrate the relationship of nursing standards to job descriptions and performance evaluations. (A further discussion of standards is presented in Chapter 2.)

The material presented in this book represents months of concentrated work, revisions, monitoring, and more revisions. A committee of nurses representing various departments and shifts in our hospitals were involved in developing and initiating the material. First, standards of nursing practice appropriate and realistic to our needs were written. Then, management personnel and all RNs and LPNs were thoroughly inserviced on the purpose, use, and meaning of the standards. Following this, the job descriptions and performance evaluations were written. (This is discussed thoroughly in Chapters 3 and 4.) Again, inservices were held for all nursing service personnel in order to acquaint them with the material. Copies of all standards, job descriptions, and performance evaluations were placed at each unit for easy access by the staff. A three-month period was allowed after introduction of the job descriptions before the new performance evaluations were actually implemented.

Once the new job descriptions and performance evaluations were put into effect, more revisions were necessary. Originally, they were too lengthy and redundant. Some items, (e.g., "good attitude") were subjective and were reworded to promote more objectivity and provide for measurement. Policies were written to support the determination of "above average" or "excellent" ratings for items on the performance evaluation, such as attendance both at work and inservice education programs. These policies also were discussed at staff meetings and thoroughly inserviced.

Management personnel were extensively inserviced in the implementation of the performance evaluations and in the collection of employee evaluation data. Time and constant feedback and monitoring were required.

Now, after about a two-year period, the new system has been proven effective. The employees are satisfied—they now know exactly what is required of them and what they must do to rate higher on their evaluations. They also show an understanding of the interrelationship among standards, job descriptions, and their performance evaluations, of the concepts behind relating these three areas, and of the necessity for doing so.

The delivery of nursing care, as defined by our standards, has improved. Now that the nurses are directly evaluated on nursing process, they are more conscious of carrying out this process throughout their practice. For example, nursing care planning previously may have included only a nursing action (such as "Give prn medication"); now it includes patient problems, desired outcomes, and nursing prescriptions. Implemented nursing actions are documented in the nurse's notes, as well as an evaluation of the action. The process or delivery of nursing care has improved, as measured against our standards of practice. The nurses are now providing the care actually defined in the standards.

The uses of this book are varied. Not only will the nurse administrator find it helpful, but additionally nurse educators and both baccalaureate and graduate degree nursing students. The material can be used by the nurse educator as a teaching aid in presenting both nursing process and systems theory and by the students to assist in understanding the relationship among standards, job descriptions, and performance evaluations, and as a guide for utilizing systems theory.

The book proceeds from an introductory chapter, giving an overview of the material, to chapters focusing on standards of nursing practice, job descriptions, and performance evaluations. A merit raise system is presented with a description of its implementation, followed by a final chapter discussing the nursing quality control system as a whole.

The last portion of the book presents detailed examples of the forms that were developed to effectively implement this system in our hospital. The forms are presented as models or guides to be used by other nursing services in developing forms consistent with the needs of their institution. This material is not presented as "the only way," but as examples found to be appropriate, realistic, and effective for our hospital. These can be easily revised and adapted for use by any organization and provide an excellent base from which to build.

In the last chapter, task-oriented job descriptions and performance evaluations are presented, such as nursing assistants, orderlies, unit secretaries, and surgical technicians. These are not directly derived from the standards as are the other job descriptions, but are presented as supplemental information for the reader.

REFERENCES

1. Joint Commission on Accreditation of Hospitals: Accreditation manual for hospitals. Chicago: Illinois, JCAH, 1981, pp. 116–117.
2. American Nurses' Association: Standards of maternal-child health nursing practice. Kansas City: Missouri, ANA, 1973.
3. American Nurses' Association: Standards of cardiovascular nursing practice. Kansas City: Missouri, ANA, 1975.
4. American Nurses' Association: Standards of nursing practice: Operating Room. Kansas City: Missouri, ANA, 1975.
5. American Nurses' Association. Standards of medical-surgical nursing practice. Kansas City: Missouri, ANA, 1974.
6. American Nurses' Association. Standards of emergency nursing practice. Kansas City: Missouri, ANA, 1975.

STANDARDS, JOB DESCRIPTIONS, AND PERFORMANCE EVALUATIONS FOR NURSING PRACTICE

1

Introduction

This chapter describes the integration of the nursing process into standards of nursing practice,* job descriptions, and performance evaluations, using a systems approach. Figure 1-1 outlines the system.

Standards, job descriptions, and performance evaluations are the components of this system. Each is a system within itself, is derived from the nursing process (see arrows, Fig. 1-1), and affects the delivery of patient care.

SYSTEMS

Systems approach is used throughout this book. Due to this fact, it deserves some explanation before the core of the material can be introduced. It is assumed that most readers have had some exposure and background in systems, so only the main points will be reviewed, leaving further in-depth discussion for books devoted entirely to the subject of systems theory. This review is by no means complete.

Ever since Ludwig von Bertalanffy's General Systems Theory[1] in the 1950s, the definition and application of a "system" has been varied. For our purposes, the definition of a system will be that it consists of interrelated parts interacting in an orderly fashion.[2] Furthermore, the parts of the system are subsystems, which consist of interrelated, interacting elements. Each subsystem is a system within itself, with the relationship of all parts together producing a meaningful whole.[3]

Some other terms associated with systems theory are input, thruput, output, and feedback. Input is the energy or information that enters the system. Thruput is the utilization and transformation of the input received, producing

---

*Unless otherwise specified, the word *standards* refers to the standards of nursing practice described in this book.

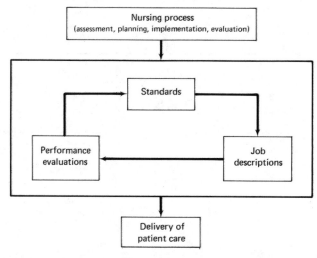

Figure 1-1   Systems approach for the nursing process.

the output. Output is the product or results of the thruput that is exported into the environment. This output reenters the system as input, and the chain of events continues. This reentering of information from the system is called feedback. Feedback can have a positive or negative effect on the system and serves as a regulator to maintain equilibrium.[4] This self-regulation involves mechanisms by which the feedback permits the system to correct itself, maintain its purpose, and continue to be effective.[5] A system must be able to regulate itself in order to maintain a steady state.[3]

If the terms input, thruput, output, and feedback were substituted into the schema presented in Fig. 1-1, they would appear as illustrated in Fig. 1-2.

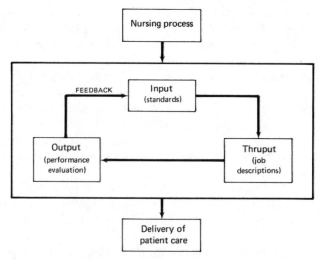

Figure 1-2   Alternate terminology for systems approach for the nursing process.

Standards are the first component of the system. They provide the input into the second component, the job descriptions. The job descriptions (thruput) transform the information received and produce the output, or third component of the system (the performance evaluation). The outcome of the performance evaluation is the final product, or results of the system, and these results feed back into the input, or standards. The output produces feedback that regulates the system. The feedback determines the effectiveness of the system and the need for adjustments, in order to maintain proper functioning.

NURSING PROCESS

The nursing process is the framework for the development of the components of our system. The definition of the nursing process is consistent with the definition of a system. It has a purpose (to provide a process to utilize for the delivery of quality nursing care), consists of interrelated components (assessment, planning, implementation, and evaluation), and the components interact in an orderly fashion (the components provide input, thruput, output, and feedback). Each component is a subsystem and can act as a separate system.[6]

The nursing process is a systematic method of assessing data, planning nursing care, implementing that care, and evaluating the effectiveness of the care.[7] It is a scientific method for problem solving, to guide the nurse's action.[8] The steps in the process are ongoing and continuous and provide for reassessment and regulation of the process, according to feedback from the evaluation phase.[7]

Assessment is the first phase of the nursing process. It is an orderly process consisting of the identification, gathering, and organization of subjective and objective data pertaining to the patient.[7] Assessment is the input phase of the nursing process.[6] It establishes baseline data concerning the health status of the patient and provides continuous information to be used in planning the patient's care.[7]

Planning is the second phase of the nursing process. It consists of determining patient present or potential problems, and desired outcomes.*[7] Planning also is the thruput phase. It transforms data collected from the assessment or input phase into meaningful arrangements, setting guidelines for the implementation phase.[6]

Implementation is the third phase of the nursing process. It is the implementation of nursing actions necessary to achieving the desired outcomes established in the planning phase. It is the nursing intervention or action taken to carry out the established plan of care.[9] Implementation is the output phase. It prescribes the action to be taken, as dictated by the planning or thruput phase, then "puts out" this prescription into action.[6]

Evaluation is the fourth phase of the nursing process. It involves determining the effectiveness of the nursing actions in achieving the plan of care.[7]

---

*The words *goal* and *desired outcome* are used interchangeably.

Evaluation includes examining patient outcomes and determining conclusions concerning the achievement or lack of achievement of desired outcomes. It involves the continual evaluation of assessment, planning, and implementation phases of the nursing process.[10] Evaluation is the feedback phase in that it directs reassessment, further planning, and revision in the total process. The information obtained by evaluation is fed back into the input or assessment phase, and this cycle continues in a systematic manner.[6] This presentation of the nursing process is basic but demonstrates the framework for which our system can be understood and utilized. (For more information concerning systems and nursing process, refer to the references and bibliography at the end of this chapter.)

A MANAGEMENT SYSTEM

It was stated earlier that a system is composed of parts that relate in such a way as to produce a meaningful whole.[3] In other words, a system must have a purpose. The purpose of the system presented in this book is to serve as a management tool in maintaining compliance with standards of nursing practice. An overview of the components of the system will be presented at this time.

The components in this management system, standards, job descriptions, and performance evaluations are derived from the nursing process. Each component is divided into four phases—assessment, planning, implementation, and evaluation. Each component utilizes these four phases in the same manner as they are used in the nursing process. For example, in the first component of the system—standards—the standards are divided into four phases. Standard I concerns assessment, Standard II concerns planning, Standard III concerns implementation, and Standard IV concerns evaluation. The same is true for the job descriptions and performance evaluations. Each is divided into the four phases of the nursing process. Then the three components, standards, job descriptions, and performance evaluations, interact as a system providing input, thruput, output, and feedback in a continuous manner, in order to achieve the purpose of maintaining the established standards of care.

Standards are the first component of the system. They are statements divided into the four phases of the nursing process, defining what is expected in the delivery of patient care. Standards define the expectations of nursing practice and delineate conditions and processes by which quality patient care can be delivered.[11] They can provide a means of measuring the quality of care delivered.[12] There are a variety of types and purposes for standards and many factors are considered in their formulation, such as patient needs, staff expertise, philosophy and goals of the institution, and quantity of available staff.[13] These and other issues will be explored in Chapter 2.

Standards must be realistic in order to be achieved. Careful assessment and planning must be done when they are formulated.[5] The assessment and planning of the standards of practice determine the expectations delineated in the job descriptions. The standards are the input that dictate the development of the job descriptions.

The content of the job descriptions is divided into the four phases of the nursing process and reflects the content of the standards of practice. Job descriptions specifically define job requirements.[13] The standards define the expectation of nursing practice and the job descriptions spell this out for the individual employee.

The job descriptions are the second component of this system. They are the thruput stage, in that they process the input from the standards into operation. They state how to implement the job in order to achieve the standards. They are the employee's contract with the institution and ensure the provision of care necessary to achieve the standards.

The performance evaluations are the third component of the system. They are the outcome or output from the implementation of the job descriptions. The performance evaluations are a mechanism by which the quality of the employee's performance is evaluated.[13] They are divided into the four phases of the nursing process and reflect the content in the job descriptions. Structured in this manner, evaluation of the employee's performance also evaluates the implementation of the job description and therefore compliance with the standards.

The outcome of the performance evaluations is also the feedback mechanism in this system. A satisfactory outcome indicates compliance with the nursing standards, whereas an unsatisfactory outcome indicates a breakdown in the system and a need for regulation. This "negative feedback" feeds back into the standards (are they realistic?) and into the job descriptions (do they clearly state the expectation?), or into other aspects of the environment that affect the system. These aspects, such as management, employee compliance and knowledge level, and other factors will be discussed in Chapter 6 concerning the quality control system.

Each component of this system has an effect upon the delivery of patient care. Standards define the type or quality of the care to be given, job descriptions specify the exact requirements in implementing that care, and the performance evaluations determine the employee's ability to deliver the care. The four phases of the nursing process are interwoven throughout each component, and each component interacts in an orderly fashion to maintain the system.

REFERENCES

1. Von Bertalanffy, L.: General systems theory. Main Currents in Modern Thought, March 1955, 11, pp. 75–83.
2. Kast, F. E., and Rosenzweig, J. E.: General systems theory: Applications for organization and management. JONA, July 1981, (11), pp. 32–41.
3. Hazzard, M. E.: An overview of systems theory. Nursing Clinics of North America, September 1971, 6(3), pp. 385–393.

4. Conway, M. E.: Clinical research: Instrument for change. JONA, December 1978, (8), pp. 27–32.

5. Bailey, J., and Claus, K.: Decision-making in nursing—Tools for change. St. Louis: C. V. Mosby Co., 1975, pp. 10–17.

6. Thompson, C.: Nursing diagnoses and defining characteristics identified of nurses practicing in primary health care settings. Unpublished dissertation. University of Alabama School of Nursing, Birmingham, 1979.

7. Yura, H., and Walsh, M.: The nursing process: Assessing, planning, implementing, evaluating. New York: Appleton-Century-Crofts, 1973.

8. Giblin, E. C.: Symposium on assessment as part of the nursing process. Nursing Clinics of North America. March 1971, 6(1), pp. 113–114.

9. Smith, S. F., and Duell, D.: Nursing skills and evaluation. Los Altos, Calif.: National Nurses' Review, 1982.

10. Gordon, M.: The concept of nursing diagnosis. Nursing Clinics of North America, September 1979, 14(3), pp. 487–496.

11. Alexanda, E. L.: Nursing administration in the hospital health care system. St. Louis: C. V. Mosby Co., 1978.

12. Miler, R. and Drake, M.: Standards of nursing performance. Tools for assuring quality care. Quality Review Bulletin, May 1980, 6(5), pp. 16–19.

13. Stevens, B.: The nurse as executive (2nd ed.). Wakefield, Mass. Nursing Resources, Inc., 1980.

BIBLIOGRAPHY

Arndt, C., and Huckabay, L.: Nursing administration theory in practice with a systems approach, (2nd ed). St. Louis: C. V. Mosby Co., 1980.

Bartas, L., and Knight, M.: Documentation of nursing process. Supervisor Nurse, January 1978, (9), pp. 42–54.

Brown, S. J.: The nursing process systems model. J. Nurs.Educ., June 1981, (20), pp. 36–40.

Bruce, J. A.: Implementation of nursing diagnosis. Nursing Clinics of North America, September 1979, 14(3), pp. 509–515.

Carrieri, V. K., and Sitzman, J.: Components of the nursing process. Nursing Clinics of North America, March 1971, 6(1), pp. 115–124.

Dossey, L.: Care giving and natural systems theory. Top Clin. Nurs., Jan. 1982, (3), pp. 21–27.

Field, L.: The implementation of nursing diagnosis in clinical practice. Nursing Clinics of North America, September 1979, 14(3), pp. 497–508.

Finley, B.: Nursing process with the battered woman. Nurse Pract., Jul/Aug. 1981, (6), pp. 11–3.

Gordon, M.: Nursing diagnoses and the diagnostic process. AJN, 1976, 16(8), pp. 1298–1300.

Hybben, L.: Systems planning smooths the way for primary nursing in a new facility. Health Serv. Manager, Jan. 1981, (14), pp. 2–4.

Kannely, J.: The meaning of evaluation. Nursing Outlook, July 1961, (9), pp. 438–440.

Kershaw, J., Lewis, M., Dale, J.: The nursing process in action. Teaching and evaluating care. A student's viewpoint (Part 2). Nurs. Times, June 1981, (77), pp. 1126–31.

Marriner, A.: The nursing process. St. Louis: C. V. Mosby Co., 1975.

McCarthy, M. M.: The nursing process. Application of current thinking in clinical problem solving. JADV Nurs., May 1981, (6), pp. 173–77.

McWilliams, C. A.: Systems analysis can solve nursing management problems. Supervisor Nurse, May 1980, (11), pp. 17–20.

Probst, M. R., Noga, J.: A decentralized nursing care delivery system. Supervisor Nurse, January 1980, (11), pp. 7–60.

Riehl, J. P., and Roy, C.: Conceptual models for practice. New York: Appleton-Century-Crofts, 1974.

Smellzer, C.: Teaching the nursing process—Practical method. J. Nurs. Educ., November 1980, (19), pp. 31–37.

Walker, L., Nicholson, R.: Criteria for evaluating nursing process models. Nurse Educator, September/October 1980, (5), pp. 8–9.

West, M. E.: Implementing effective nursing staffing systems in the managed hospital. Top Health Care Financ., Summer 1980, (6), pp. 11–25.

2

Standards of Nursing Practice

QUALITY ASSURANCE

Before delving into the subject of standards of practice, it is necessary to first understand the general concept of quality assurance. Throughout the literature, this term has been defined in a variety of ways, and the meaning can be confusing to the reader. The following explanation is the interpretation of quality assurance that is used in this book.

According to Zimmer,[1] quality assurance encompasses necessary changes or improvements to ensure survival. It involves identifying standards for excellence, evaluating care against those standards, and then taking action to correct deficiencies and achieve the standards. The assurance of quality care can only be achieved by continual evaluation and follow-up corrective actions.

Schmadl[2] states that quality assurance is assuring excellence. He defines excellence as a variable on a continuum that will differ from institution to institution, or person to person. He states that excellence is a value judgment made by the health care providers, with many factors being considered, such as the type of institutions and the consumer.

Slee[3] has identified three necessary elements in a quality assurance program: standards, surveillance, and corrective action. In order to assure quality, standards must first be established, or the definition of excellence. Then the standards are monitored and evaluated for achievement, and feedback from the evaluation is utilized for corrective action.

Formulation of Standards

Formulation of standards is the first step toward evaluating the nursing care delivery. The standards serve as a base by which the quality of care can be judged. This judgment may be according to a rating, or other data that reflect the conformity of existing practice with the established standards.[4] The standards must be written, regularly reviewed, and well-known by the nursing staff.[3]

STRUCTURE—PROCESS—OUTCOME

Standards can be established to appraise care according to many approaches. The most common approaches are based on structure, process, and outcome.[5] The nursing organization or structure is usually evaluated according to structure standards, the activities or delivery of care are evaluated by process standards, and the patient's status is evaluated by outcome standards. But all three types of standards are interrelated and can be used to evaluate various aspects in a nursing service.[6]

A structure standard involves the "setup" of the institution. The philosophy, goals and objectives, structure of the organization, facilities and equipment, and qualifications of the employees are some of the components of the structure of the organization. A process standard involves the activities concerned with delivering patient care. These standards measure nursing actions, or lack of actions, involving patient care. An outcome standard measures the patient's change in health status. This change may be due to nursing care, medical care, or as a result of a variety of services offered to the patient.[2] Outcome standards reflect effectiveness and results, rather than the process of giving the care.[6]

When formulating standards, one must decide on the definition of excellence and the method by which to evaluate the excellence (i.e., structure, process, or outcome). The definition of excellence may be consistent with pre-existing standards, such as the ANA's standards of nursing practice, or it may be standards developed according to one's own philosophy and values. The authors advocate the use of the ANA's standards, either in their entirety or in an adapted form as presented in this book.

As for the method for evaluating excellence, all three processes can be involved when constructing standards, or simply one, such as outcome. If the results, or outcome only, are to be evaluated, then the standards are constructed in such a way as to measure the outcome or alteration in the patient's health status.

For example, in a newly postoperative colostomy patient, a nursing outcome standard might be stated as: Patient will demonstrate self-irrigation using the routine and equipment that will be used at home.[7] Many approaches and methods to standard formulation and validation are being implemented. Refer to the references and bibliography at the end of this chapter for some of the current literature in this area.

The standards presented in this book are constructed in such a way as to mainly evaluate excellence according to process. Schmadl states that no one of the three approaches to evaluation is a valid indicator of quality of care, but only when structure, process, and outcome are all involved is quality of care actually measured.[2] The authors of this book agree with this and promote the management system presented in this book as one means of contributing to the evaluation of nursing care. We also encourage further study and research to validate this system by its comparison with actual patient outcomes.

ANA's STANDARDS OF PRACTICE

Despite the definition of quality as being an individual judgment, it is important to formulate standards based on valid and sound principles. That is why the utilization or adaptation of the ANA's standards of practice are advocated, as they were developed by nursing professionals with expert knowledge of nursing practice. That is also why all aspects of the nursing process were incorporated into this system, as the nursing process has been universally accepted by nursing experts as a framework for nursing practice.[8]

Originally in this system, the ANA standards of nursing practice were adapted as the nursing standards in all areas of nursing service. But after inservicing and staff meetings, the nurses expressed confusion and concern over some of the statements in the stadards. For instance, the nurses became "hung up" on the term, *nursing diagnosis,*[9] and had much apprehension over what was being expected of them. Most of their emphasis was being placed on the terminology, rather than the process of assessment and problem identification. They were concerned over what they must *change* or do differently concerning their patient care, in order to make a "nursing diagnosis."

The majority of the nurses in this institution were diploma and associate degree graduates of at least 10 years. This was a factor that influenced our changing the wording in the standards. They had difficulty grasping the new terms and too much time was being spent teaching the terms for many processes the nurses were already practicing. It was not that the terms were unimportant, but rather that the necessity of understanding the "process" was most important, and the newness of the terms had invoked an obstacle to the learning of this process.

So a committee was formed to revise the nursing standards and to assist in initiating the new standards into our nursing service. The Medical-Surgical Standards of Nursing Practice were written first; then these were used as a guide for writing the standards for the other nusing departments. The following is the rationale for revising the ANA standards into the ones presented in this book. (Refer to the Standards of Medical-Surgical Nursing Practice, Chapter 7.)

REVISION OF THE NURSING STANDARDS

First of all, because the nursing process was to be integrated into our system for nursing practice, it was decided that the standards should be divided into the four phases of assessment, planning, implementation, and evaluation. This provided a clearer correlation with the job descriptions and performance evaluations, which were also to be divided into the four phases of the nursing process. It reinforced acceptance of nursing process as a framework for the practice of nursing and promoted understanding of the relationship among the standards, job descriptions, and performance evaluations.

For Standard I, the Committe wanted very specific criteria. They listed all elements they felt were essential to a comprehensive patient history and physical, and these became the criteria for asessment. Standard I of the ANA's Medical-Surgical Nursing Practice[9] was studied carefully. Some assessment factors that we felt could not be easily documented for evaluation, like growth and development, were omitted. Again, this is not because these factors are unimportant, but that they could not be realistically documented and evaluated in our institution. This fact was determined from the initial trial period of the ANA standards. Other than omitting some items, others were combined or reworded to facilitate understanding by the nurses. The word *patient* instead of *client* was chosen due to the fact that the nurses felt more comfortable using this term.

Standard II became the planning stage. According to Yura and Walsh,[8] planning begins with nursing diagnoses and ends with the development of the plan of care. The ANA Standards II and III were combined into our Standard II. Again, after deliberation over terminology best suited to our nursing service's needs, the words *patient problems* were substituted for *nursing diagnoses*. Even though nursing diagnoses encompass a broader definition than *present or potential patient problems,* the committee decided on this term. In inservicing the standards, the definition of present/potential patient problems was communicated consistently with the accepted definition of a nursing diagnosis. It was simply by substituting the words that better acceptance and understanding was achieved.

The same was true with the words *goals* and *desired outcomes*. The existing Kardexes, with which the nurses were presently writing care plans, had the titles of Patient Problems, Desired Outcomes, and Prescribed Nursing Actions at the top in three columns. They had been previously instituted when teaching care planning, and there was no need to introduce an additional unnecessary change when the words actually had the same meaning. The nurses were already comfortable with thinking of desired outcomes as the patient's goal. Therefore, the committee decided to substitute the terms *desired outcome* for *goals* throughout the standards.

The committee also decided to add additional criteria to the planning stage of Standard II. This was the incorporation of home health care into the desired outcome. The nurses felt that this was important enough to warrant being separated and given special emphasis, and that planning for home health care must be initiated following the initial assessment of the patient on admission.

For Standard III the committee combined the ANA's standards concerning nursing prescriptions and nursing actions into one standard. This one standard involves the implementation stage of the nursing process. The nurses felt that the prescription and resulting implementation of nursing actions should be under the same section. Again, certain items as presented by the ANA were omitted, combined, or reworded, but the concepts and meanings were kept the same.

The last standard concerns the evaluation phase of the nursing process. The committee decided that in order to promote understanding of the word *evaluation* this should be combined into one standard. Despite the fact that reassessment and revision of the nursing care plan involve separate nursing actions, they both are a result of the evaluation process and are directed by the data collected from evaluation. The criteria for Standard IV, evaluation, were established from Standard VII and VIII of the ANA's Standards of Nursing Practice.[10]

The next step following the formulation of the standards of nursing practice is a thorough clarification of the meaning of each standard.

CLARIFICATION OF EACH STANDARD

Standard I

Standard I, assessment, is described as the identification and gathering of data concerning the health status of the patient. This process must be complete, or thorough, continuous, or ongoing, and systematic, or performed in a scientific manner. The achievement of this standard is measured by the achievement of the descriptive criteria under the standard. In other words, when the criteria are achieved, the assessment standard is met. The criteria are grouped into five categories and, when put together, comprise a definition of what is considered a quality assessment.

The first category under assessment is a *comprehensive patient history and physical*. According to the standard, for a history and physical to be comprehensive it should include the patient interview, psychological assessment, physical assessment, as well as the patient's perception of his illness.[11] Only when these are completely and accurately assessed is a comprehensive history and physical completed, and therefore one portion of the overall Standard I, assessment.

In referring to the Standards of Medical-Surgical Nursing Practice in Chapter 7, it can be seen that there are 11 items listed under Patient Interview. These items are the criteria necessary to complete a thorough interview. Each item or criterion must be documented in some manner in order to be met. A nursing interview or assessment form is helpful in meeting assessment criteria, and a sample of such a form is presented in Fig. 2-1. This form ensures that all initial data are collected in accordance with Standard I in a complete and systematic manner. Documentation of the continual patient assessment is evidenced in the nurses' notes and on the nursing care plan, as will be discussed later.

The following is a description of all criteria under category one, a comprehensive patient history and physical. Each criterion is defined according to its meaning and how it is documented on the nursing interview and assessment form (Fig. 2-1).

SOUTH BALDWIN HOSPITAL
Foley, Alabama

Nursing Interview and Assessment

Admission date_____ Time_____

Mode of arrival_____

ID bracelet: Yes____ No_____

Height_____ Weight_____

BP_____ Lt/Rt Pulse_____

Respiration_____

Temp.   Oral/Rectal/Axillary

HEALTH HISTORY:

Chief complaint:_____

_____

Further description of chief
complaint:_____

_____

_____

PAIN:
Location:_____

_____

Character: Sharp ( ) Dull ( )
Constant ( ) Intermittent ( )

Relief measures:_____

_____

_____

PERTINENT MEDICAL AND SURGICAL
HISTORY: _____

_____

_____

_____

FAMILY HISTORY:

Diabetes	Yes	No
Hypertension	Yes	No
TB	Yes	No
Anemia	Yes	No
Cancer	Yes	No
Heart disease	Yes	No
Mental illness	Yes	No
Rheumatic fever	Yes	No

COMMENTS: _____

_____

_____

INFORMATION FOR INTERVIEW:
Obtained from:
Patient ___ Family member _____
Other (Name)_____

_____

ALLERGIES:
Drugs:_____

_____

Other:_____

_____

MEDICATIONS USED AT HOME: (Prescription/nonprescription)

Name	Dosage	Frequency	Last taken	Reason	If med here
____	____	____	____	____	____
____	____	____	____	____	____
____	____	____	____	____	____
____	____	____	____	____	____
____	____	____	____	____	____

Sent to pharmacy( ) Not brought to hosp.( ) Sent home ( )
To pharmacy for ID ( )

PERSONAL DATA:
Home diet:
Appetite:
Restrictions:
Food and fluid preferences:

_____

HABITS/PREFERENCES:
Use of alcohol   Yes No
How much_____
Use of tobacco   Yes No
Type/how much_____

Sleeping aids   Yes No

Rt/Lt handed _____
Diversion/Hobbies_____

Personal hygiene/grooming

Nutritional status: obese ( )
thin( ) emaciated( ) normal( )
ADL consistent with age Yes No
(If No, comment_____

Attending physician notified
Yes_____ Time_____
ORIENTATION TO ROOM:
( )Nurse call light( )Bathroom
( )Bed controls   ( )TV
( )Meal time   ( )Phone
( )Visiting hours ( )Smoking
( )Thermostat   policy
( )Bed lock   ( )Side rail
( )Hosp. booklet   policy
( )Recommended rubber
   soled slippers

VALUABLES STATEMENT: I have
been advised to take all valuables to business office safe
or send them home. I accept
responsibility for anything I
keep at my bedside.

Signature:_____
List of valuables:_____

_____

Disposition of valuables:

_____

Witness:_____

PROSTHESIS:

Dentures: Upper	Yes	No
Lower	Yes	No
Removable bridge	Yes	No
Artificial eye	Yes	No
Contact lens	Yes	No
Glasses	Yes	No
Hearing aid	Yes	No
Pacemaker	Yes	No
Artificial limbs	Yes	No
Brace	Yes	No
Wig	Yes	No

Explanation:_____

Figure 2-1 Sample nursing interview and assessment form. (*Continued.*)

REVIEW OF SYSTEMS

HEENT
Hearing disturbances	Yes	No
Vision disturbances	Yes	No
Nosebleeds	Yes	No
Speech deficit	Yes	No
Difficulty swallowing	Yes	No
Unequal pupils	Yes	No
Disequilibrium	Yes	No
Drainage	Yes	No

Comments:

RESPIRATORY
Irregular	Yes	No
Shallow	Yes	No
Dyspnea	Yes	No
Orthopnea	Yes	No
Cough	Yes	No

Sputum:

Breath sounds:
Adventitious	Yes	No
Unequal	Yes	No
Absent	Yes	No
Chest asymmetry	Yes	No

Comments:

CARDIOVASCULAR
Edema	Yes	No
Arrhythmias	Yes	No
Varicosities	Yes	No

Peripheral pulses:
Weak	Yes	No
Unequal	Yes	No
Absent	Yes	No

Comments:

SKIN
Petechial	Yes	No
Hot	Yes	No
Cold	Yes	No
Scaly/dry	Yes	No
Diaphoretic	Yes	No

Color:
Pale	Yes	No
Cyanotic	Yes	No
Flushed	Yes	No
Amputation	Yes	No
(Limb)		
Ostomy	Yes	No
(Site)		
Skin abnormalities	Yes	No

Comments:

CHEST
Breast:
Discharge	Yes	No
Bleeding	Yes	No
Nipple retraction	Yes	No
Last breast exam:		

Comments:

GASTROINTESTINAL
Nausea/vomiting	Yes	No
Recent weight loss/gain	Yes	No
Distention	Yes	No
Tarry stools	Yes	No
Hard abdomen	Yes	No
Tender abdomen	Yes	No
Diarrhea	Yes	No
Constipation	Yes	No

Bowel sounds:
Hypoactive	Yes	No
Hyperactive	Yes	No
Absent	Yes	No
Last bowel movement:		

Comments:

MUSCULOSKELETAL
Back pain	Yes	No
Neck pain	Yes	No
Extremity pain	Yes	No
Joint swelling	Yes	No
Fractures	Yes	No
Range of motion:		

Comments:

GENITOURINARY
Dysuria	Yes	No
Frequency	Yes	No
Burning	Yes	No
Nocturia	Yes	No
Hematuria	Yes	No
Incontinence	Yes	No
Retention	Yes	No

Comments:

Male:
| Prostate problems | Yes | No |

Comments:

Female:
LMP
| Vaginal discharge | Yes | No |
| Unusual vag. bleeding | Yes | No |

Comments:

MENTAL/NEUROLOGICAL
Syncope	Yes	No
Seizure	Yes	No
Restlessness	Yes	No
Dizziness	Yes	No
Headache	Yes	No
Paralysis	Yes	No
Lethargic	Yes	No
Semicomatose	Yes	No
Comatose	Yes	No
Confused	Yes	No

Comments:

EMOTIONAL STATUS AND PATTERNS OF COPING
Depressed	Yes	No
Crying	Yes	No
Nervous	Yes	No
Withdrawn	Yes	No

Other:

Barriers identified that prevent learning home care instr.

Cultural, socio/economic and environmental conditions pertinent to health care

Additional information:

Concerns during hospitalization

Patient's desired outcome from hospitalization

Sig. of nurse assessing patient:

RN assessment signature:

Time:

Figure 2-1(*Continued*) Systems review.

Patient interview:

Chief complaint. The reason patient has sought medical attention, preferably stated in patient's own words. This is written briefly, using one word or a sentence.[11]

History of present illness. A further description of chief complaint (i.e., when problem began, how it progressed, etc.). It also involves a description of any pain, including the location, character, and any relief measures.[11]

Allergies. Any drug allergies or adverse side effects to drugs would be documented under this category. Any food allergies or allergies to dust, mold, or other inhalants could also be documented as "other."

Medications. This includes any prescription or nonprescription medications used at home. Documentation should include the name, dosage, frequency, time medication was last taken, reason for taking the medication, and whether the medication was brought to the hospital. If the patient does not know what the medication is, it is sent to the pharmacy for identification. No medicines are kept at the bedside unless specifically ordered by the physician, and, if so, they must be identified by the pharmacy. The family should take the medicines home, following the assessment, or if that is not possible, they are kept in the pharmacy until the patient is discharged.

Past medical history. This section includes only pertinent medical (and surgical) history that is related to the patient's hospitalization. Documenting a tonsillectomy at age 6 for an 86-year-old patient would not be necessary. Brevity is indicated so that the nurse is not compelled to document lengthy past history that is repeated by the physician and other health care workers. Family History is also covered under this section, where the nurse assesses whether the patient has a family history of diabetes, hypertension, tuberculosis, anemia, cancer, heart disease, mental illness, or rheumatic fever. All data in the past history as well as the other assessment categories are used for problem identification and care planning.

Cultural and socioeconomic conditions. (See second page of Fig. 2-1, right column.) Throughout the assessment, the nurse collects data, either by questions or observation, that are pertinent to the patient's health care. Any customs, special beliefs and practices, or social and economic or environmental conditions that would affect the patient's health care or hospitalization[12] should be identified and documented. An example of this would be a newly diagnosed diabetic patient who is a migrant worker. There are special socioeconomic and environmental conditions that need to be identified and documented so that proper planning can be done for the patient's discharge. Teaching for self-care would be altered to consider the special "home" conditions.

Activities of daily living. This section includes activities that the patient performs concerning bathing, brushing teeth, combing hair, and in general "doing for himself." It is the patient's capacity for self-care.[13] The nurse assesses whether the activities of daily living (ADL) are consistent with the patient's age and, if not, documents an explanation.

Personal habits. An assessment of personal habits is completed that includes use of alcohol, tobacco, sleeping aids, and personal diversions and hobbies.[11]

Food and fluid preferences. This section includes home diet, descriptions of the patient's usual appetite at home, any restrictions to diet, and special food and fluid preferences.

Appetite changes/weight changes. This is assessed and documented in two different sections. Appetite is addressed under personal data concerning the above food and fluid preferences. On the second page of Fig. 2-1, under gastrointestinal assessment, the nurse determines whether the patient has experienced any recent weight loss or gain and documents this.

Available and accessible human, community, and material resources. This is an assessment of what the patient has in the way of support systems at home, agencies to assist with home care, supplies and equipment or materials needed for home care. It involves persons or resources necessary to optimal health care at home. The nurse identifies those resources pertinent to the patient's health care and documents them in the designated section. This is from the initial assessment, of course, and, as the nurse gathers additional information throughout the patient's hospitalization, she may identify further resources necessary for the patient's home care. These would be added to the care plan and documented in the nurses' notes.

In addition to the patient interview, a psychological assessment is completed in order to obtain a comprehensive patient history and physical. Under a psychological assessment, there are three criteria. The first two, emotional status and pattern of coping, are assessed and documented together. This is done because of the interrelatedness of the two and to facilitate documentation. On the assessment form, they are broken down into assessing whether the patient is depressed, crying, nervous, withdrawn, or exhibiting any other unusual behavior. This assesses and documents the emotional status and patterns of coping in "negatives." In other words, if the patient is not depressed, or crying, or nervous, or withdrawn, or any other condition, he is calm and coping well with his hospitalization. The nurses decided that these five areas would allow for the documentation of any problems involved with the patient's emotional status and coping, and that if it was not documented there was no problem in this area. That way the assessment can be thorough and even quite lengthy, where the documentation is simple and concise.

Concerns during hospitalization. This involves exactly what it says. Anything that the patient may be concerned with during the hospitalization should be documented. For example, if the patient is a single parent and has no one to keep her child at home, she would definitely be concerned about this and it would be a problem. This should be documented on the assessment form and integrated into the patient's care plan. Often these concerns are immediate needs that the nurse must address and for which she must seek solutions.

The next major section under category one is the physical assessment. This includes the personal hygiene and grooming, nutritional status, mental status, and physical status. These are described and documented in the following manner:

Personal hygiene and grooming. This includes, in general, the patient's cleanliness and gives clues to many other aspects of the patient's health status. An assessment is done, observing the patient throughout the physical assessment and interview, determining body cleanliness, neatness of appearance, grooming of hair, etc. A statement summing up this assessment is documented in the appropriate place.

Nutritional status. This is an assessment of whether the patient is obese, thin, emaciated, or normal. These categories sum up the various types of nutritional status and ease documentation.

Mental status. This section encompasses two areas. One is combined with a neurological assessment and involves problems ranging from restlessness to confusion. The other area concerns the patient's ability to understand. An assessment of the mental status is done throughout the entire initial history and physical, and the nurse determines the patient's ability to comprehend and learn necessary information for home care.[11] This is assessed and any problems or barriers to learning are identified and documented so that if family members or agencies need to be involved, this can be identified early and included in the care plan.[14]

Physical status. The nurse's assessment of the patient's physical status is documented under the section called "Review of Systems." Some of this section involves questions, and some involves observation, inspection, auscultation, and palpation. The systems are divided mainly into HEENT (head, eyes, ears, nose, and throat), Respiratory, Cardiovascular, Skin, Chest, Gastrointestinal, Musculoskeletal, Mental/Neurological, and Genitourinary. Some additional assessment areas are included, such as last menstrual period for the female and prostate problems for the male. Notice that the format is set up in such a way as to identify problems. For instance, does the patient have hearing disturbances? A "yes" or "no" is circled, and, if "yes," then an appropriate comment must be made. This way the sheet can be easily scanned at a later date and any problems marked yes are easily identified. This also assists in problem identification to initiate the patient's plan of care. It helps the nurse focus in on abnormalities and areas in need of correction or attention.

The items under the review of systems are a combination of the most frequent problems encountered and seem to encompass as comprehensive a physical assessment as possible. For example, hearing disturbances are problems that would involve deafness, tinnitus, and any other condition involving hearing. This way it is grouped into one item, and, if it is a problem, an explanatory comment is made.

Perception of illness is the last area comprising category one, comprehensive patient history and physical. It is how the patient sees and understands his health status.[12] The nurse assesses the patient's understanding of the disease/illness and reasons for hospitalization throughout the assessment. The patient's desired outcome from hospitalization indicates his perception of his illness. By documenting the desired outcomes, the patient's understanding is also reflected. For example, a patient with chronic obstructive lung disease is admitted to the hospital with extreme dyspnea. He has had this disease for 15 years and has progressively become weakened and unable to perform activities of daily living. After being hospitalized and assessed, he verbalizes that he expects to stay here long enough this time to recover and be able to play golf again. From this statement he reveals many things, from patterns of coping and defense mechanisms to perception of illness. The nurse can delve into these areas to determine the problem. The patient's statement also reflects a lack of understanding of the progressive and limiting nature of the disease and the real reasons for hospitalization. So by obtaining the patient's desired outcome from hospitalization, much information can be obtained. For practicality and space purposes, only desired outcome is documented on the assessment form. But the nurse transfers information concerning the patient's understanding of reasons for hospitalization and the disease process/illness to the nurses' notes and care plan to be used later for patient teaching.

The second of the five categories of criteria under Standard I is *the collection of data from available sources*. According to the standard, for data to be collected from available sources, it should include patient, family, significant other health care providers, and individuals and/or agencies in the community. This means that all possible sources should be investigated for information concerning the patient. For example, if a patient was transferred from a nursing home, a patient history should be obtained from those nurses, with any information concerning the needs of the patient. Documentation of this would be listed under "Additional information" on the interview form, and the name and title of the person supplying the information would be listed under "information obtained from." A notation in the nurses' notes may also be necessary. Only when data are collected from all possible sources can a thorough assessment be completed, and the assessment standard be met.

The third category of criteria under Standard I concerns *the collection of data by scientific methodology*. This means that data are collected in a scientific and systematic manner, using all available techniques. Data are collected by interview, observation, inspection, auscultation, palpation, and reports and records. Interview involves talking to the patient, family, etc. and asking questions.[12] Observation concerns observing the patient's affect, skin, reactions, and physical characteristics while interviewing or performing the review of systems.[15] Inspection is actively looking at the patient and seeking specific signs and symptoms or abnormalities while doing the review of systems.[11] Auscultation is listening with a stethoscope, such as listening for heart sounds.[11] Palpation is the act of feeling with the hands. It is applying the fingers with light pressure to the body to determine what is beneath. It is also used for determining tenderness or pain.[11] Collection of data from reports and records would involve lab reports, old charts, nursing notes, progress notes, or the care plan. Anything in the way of a written report would be included here.

The collection of data using the above methods is documented on the interview form and in the nurses' notes. For instance, by circling "yes" next to adventitious breath sounds on the interview form would indicate an assessment by auscultation. By a statement in the nurses' notes concerning notifying the physician of a low hemoglobin report, an assessment was made from reports and records.

The fourth category under the assessment standard concerns the *organization of data in a systematic arrangement*. Data must be organized in order to have a complete, continuous, and systematic assessment performed. The arrangement of data must provide for accurate collection, complete collection, accessibility, and confidentiality. All four of these criteria must be met in order for the data to be systematically organized and to therefore meet Standard I.

Management plays a large part in meeting these criteria by ensuring that the institution allows for organization of the data. An accurate and complete collection of data must be collected by the nurse, but the assessment form must be organized in such a way as to facilitate this. In other words, the form provides for completeness by including all necessary items. Its wording is such that accuracy in data collection is enhanced. The structure of the nurses' station and charting system would determine the accessibility of the data collection. If nurses' notes are kept in separate locations from the rest of the chart, it might be more difficult to get a complete assessment from all sources. Also, policy and procedure development and enforcement would facilitate the achievement of these criteria.

The accuracy and completeness of data collection are evidenced in the nurses' notes, on the interview form, and on the care plans. Confidentiality is evidenced by observation of the nurse's conduct, and simply listening. Accessibility, though largely a management responsibility, can be evidenced by the appropriate forms, reports, etc. being placed in the proper location. All four of these criteria must be carried out for the arrangement of data to be organized in such a manner as to facilitate a proper and complete assessment.

The fifth and last category under Standard I is the *communication of data in an orderly fashion*. Communication of data is crucial for a continuous, complete, and systematic assessment to be obtained. Data are any information concerning the patient, and, in order to be useful, they must be shared. For communication to be orderly, it must meet four criteria. The first is that the data are recorded by each shift, daily. That simply means each shift the nurses' notes reflect data collected concerning the patient. The second is that data are updated each shift, daily. This means that any new data collected must be added to the nurses' notes and care plan each shift. As problems are solved and progress is made, an updated assessment is documented. Updated data are added each shift, daily, to the nurses' notes. The third criterion is that data are revised and recorded as appropriate. This means that new problems identified, changes in the plan of care, new reports, or change in actions taken are all documented when they occur. All of the above three criteria involve simply the documentation of patient status, progress, and the present plan of care daily by each shift. The fourth criterion is that all of this must be communicated verbally among the health team daily. This communicating involves a nurses' report between shifts, reporting assessment data to the physician, or discussion of the patient's health status and plan with another department, such as physical therapy. Whatever is assessed concerning the patient must be documented and communicated.

Standard II

Standard II is the planning standard. It consists of determining the patient's problems and desired outcomes and initiating planning for home care. The achievement of this standard is determined by meeting the criteria listed under the three categories, identification of patient problems, formulation of desired outcomes, and incorporation of home health care into the desired outcomes.

The first category, *identification of present/potential patient problems,* stems from the patient assessment. As listed in the criteria, the data collected from the assessment must first be grouped into meaningful arrangements, based upon scientific knowledge. This is "making some sense" out of lab values, physical findings, and other assessment data. Once the data are grouped into meaningful arrangements, the patient's health status is determined. This is then compared to the norms to determine present or potential problems. This is similar to making a nursing diagnosis. What the criteria are defining are the thought processes taken in order to gather data and arrive at identified patient problems. The patient's health status and problems are documented in the nurses' notes and on the care plan. But problems must be identified in the sequence listed in the criteria in order for the planning standard to be achieved. Once the problems are identified, they must be given priority according to their impact upon the patient's health status. If a patient has high blood pressure of 200/100, this problem would have to be approached before his problem of lack of knowledge concerning salt-free diet. The order of priority is documented on the care plan so that corresponding desired outcomes can be formulated.

Once the problems are identified and given priority, *desired outcomes are formulated.* This is the second category under the planning standard. Desired outcomes are formulated when all the criteria listed below it are met.

The first criterion under desired outcomes is that the patient (family, significant other) and nurse mutually agree upon the health problems. In other words, the patient/family must agree that there is a problem and what it is. For example, it would be unrealistic to expect a diabetic patient to inject his own insulin if he is denying that he is diabetic. So the problem of top priority would be the patient's denial. The nurse would work with the patient in simply identifying denial as a problem. This agreement would be documented in the nurse's notes.

The second criterion is that the patient and nurse mutually agree upon the desired outcomes. From the problem of denial mentioned above, the desired outcome would be acceptance of the diagnosis of diabetes. The patient and nurse must mutually agree on this goal in order to make progress. These first two criteria stress the importance of participation and involvement of patients and families in planning of health care. The nurses' notes would reflect this participation.

The third criterion under formulation of desired outcomes is that they are congruent with the patient problems and established norms. First of all, the goal must correspond to the problem. If the problem is anxiety, the desired outcome should concern reducing this anxiety, or in some way reflect the problem, and not some other problem. Also, norms must be considered. It would be unrealistic to set a goal outside of normal range. For instance, if a patient is short of breath, a desired outcome written on the care plan may read, "Within 8 hours the respirations will be between 12 and 20." Knowledge of normal respirations is necessary, so that the goal is realistic.

The fourth criterion is that the desired outcomes be specific. This does not mean "relieve signs and symptoms" or "restore to optimal functioning." A specific desired outcome states exactly what is expected. "Within 8 hours the patient will show no signs of anxiety, such as wringing hands, constant talking, restlessness," would be a good example.

Desired outcomes are measurable within a certain time frame. This is the fifth criterion. This means simply that they must be measurable in order to be evaluated. A desired outcome, such as "The patient will ambulate," does not provide a means to measure its achievement. It should be written as "6/29 at 8 a.m. the patient will ambulate from the bathroom back to the bed." This states exactly what is expected.

Desired outcomes are consistent with other health providers' expectations. This is the sixth criterion. In other words, nurses' goals and plans of care should not conflict with medical care or other health care providers' goals. If respiratory therapy's desired outcome is to increase the oxygen level and decrease the carbon dioxide level in the patient's blood gases, nursing's goals should coincide. The desired outcomes might involve turning, conserving energy, providing oxygen, and many other actions necessary to help oxygenate the patient. The nurse's desired outcome might be written "Within 8 hours the patient will exhibit no signs of cyanosis at nail beds or around lips," for a problem identified as cyanosis. This criterion identifies the importance of nursing working with all other health providers, agreeing on the problems, and setting similar goals so that they are all working toward the same outcome.

Whereas the desired outcome on the plan of care must be amenable to nursing actions,[8] it should be consistent with the medical diagnosis. If a patient is diagnosed as diabetic, the identified patient problem might involve the patient's lack of knowledge concerning the disease process.

The seventh and last criterion under desired outcomes is that they are established to restore the patient's optimal functioning capabilities. This means that goals must be individualized for each patient to help him obtain the best health status possible. Age, physical condition, educational level, and other factors affect optimal functioning, but the nurse strives toward the optimal for each patient. This is not written as a goal but is determined by the assessment and used as a guide in setting desired outcomes. Patient abilities vary, and what is realistic for one patient would not be for another. One would not set the same goals for a paraplegic as a nonparaplegic. That is what this criterion is all about.

The third category of criterion under the planning standard concerns home health care. Planning for discharge is begun immediately following the initial assessment, and desired outcomes include the incorporation of home health care. This means that teaching is planned concerning: (1) disease processes and complications, (2) medication, (3) diet, (4) exercise/activity, (5) self-care techniques and materials, and (6) available support systems and resources. The assessment is the gathering of baseline data. Then problems concerning home care are identified and desired outcomes are formulated with the patient/family concerning the six areas listed. The problem and desired outcome are written on the care plan, the teaching and patient's learning are documented on the nurses' notes. Special teaching and discharge summary forms are often used to facilitate the communication and documentation of learning. According to the standard, home health care must be incorporated in some way into every patient's plan of care. Only by meeting the criteria listed under identification of the patient's problem, formulation of desired outcomes, and incorporating home health care into desired outcomes can Standard II be achieved.

Standard III

The third standard is the implementation stage of the Medical-Surgical Standards of Nursing Practice. It reads: "The plan of care is implemented in order to achieve the desired outcome." The plan of care must be put into action, or implemented, in order to achieve the desired outcome. The implementation standard is achieved when the two categories of criteria listed below it are met.

The first category consists of the *formulation of nursing prescriptions that delineate actions to be taken*. Nursing prescriptions are nursing orders that prescribe what is to be done—and *HOW*. They are written statements that spell out the exact action to be implemented.[8] They are written on the care plan and followed by each shift, day to day, in order to implement the nursing actions in a consistent manner. In formulating nursing prescriptions, certain principles must be recognized and utilized. These principles are listed as the critera under category 1, formulation of prescriptions.

1. Nursing prescriptions are specific to the identified patient problems and desired outcomes. This simply means that the actions prescribed must relate to the problem and goal. On the nursing care plan, if the problem is identified as shortness of breath, the desired outcome may read: "Within 4 hours the patient's respirations will be between 12 and 20 per minute." The nursing prescriptions written on the care plan would read something like: "Increase head of bed 45 degrees, place small pillow behind back between shoulder blades, keep room tidy and articles within easy reach, and noise to a minimum," etc. These prescribed actions relate to the problem and desired outcome.

2. Prescribed actions are based on current scientific knowledge. Nursing actions prescribed must be based on accepted nursing practice that has been proven to be effective. For instance, an immobilized patient is known to have the possibility of developing pneumonia. Certain actions, like turning frequently from side to side, taking deep breaths, range of motion to increase circulation, and other actions have been proven effective in decreasing the chances of pneumonia. This is what is meant by being "based on current scientific knowledge."

3. Prescribed actions incorporate principles of patient teaching. This may involve anything from orientation to the hospital and the patient room to cardiac rehabilitation. Patient teaching is an important aspect of the patient's care. On every care plan, teaching should enter into some aspect of the patient's care. So knowledge of theory and principles of patient teaching is necessary for nurses. Nurses must incorporate identifying the need for teaching, patient readiness, patient motivation, barriers to learning, types of learning, and use of taxonomies in teaching the patients.[14]

4. Prescribed actions incorporate principles of psychosocial interactions. If the nurse is aware of the psychological adaptations made by patients during hospitalizations and the resulting social reactions, she will be more able to meet the patient's needs and implement the plan of care. For instance, in patient teaching, nursing prescriptions must take into account the level of acceptance the patient has obtained toward his illness, thus identifying the appropriate time to begin teaching. The patient's psychosocial adaptation to his illness will determine his ability to learn. Redman[14] discusses this process of adaptation and the need for appropriate nursing support and understanding to help guide the patient through the various stages. The nurse can time her teaching according to the patient's acceptance and readiness to learn.

5. Prescribed actions incorporate environmental factors influencing the patient's health. Again referring to patient teaching, certain environmental factors play a large part in accomplishing desired outcomes. For instance, in writing nursing prescriptions concerning teaching the patient about certain aspects of his illness, factors like privacy, noise control, warm and accepting atmosphere, and physical comfort all contribute to learning.[14] The environment must be considered in the formulation of all prescriptions, so that the patient will feel safe, secure, free from interruptions, and have a minimum of noise.

6. Appropriate human material and community resources must be incorporated into nursing prescriptions. From the assessment, baseline data

are collected concerning the patient's suport systems, need for assistance by agencies, necessary supplies and equipment needed for home care. On the care plan, actions are prescribed to fulfill the needs identified, and to ensure that steps are taken to get the necessary resources. For example, in prescribing actions concerning teaching of colostomy irrigation, the prescriptions would include involving family member or support person, ensuring that the appropriate equipment is available and accessible to the patient after discharge, and making sure the local ostomy agency is contacted and available for questions and support.

7. Prescribed actions include keeping the patient knowledgeable of his health status and total health care plan. When a patient is kept informed of his status and progress, he can be more involved in his care. Because the patient participates in problem identification and goal setting, it is necessary that he be knowledgeable of his status and the total health care plan. This would be written on the care plan, for example, by prescribing measures to tell the patient his progress toward achievement of desired outcomes, explaining the necessity for certain procedures, and explaining the overall plan of care.

The second category of criteria for Standard III concerns the *implementation of actions delineated in the nursing prescriptions*. The criteria listed state that the actions implemented must: (1) involve the patient/family, (2) be consistent with the nursing prescriptions, (3) be based on current scientific knowledge, (4) be flexible and individualized for each patient, (5) include principles of safety, and (6) include principles of infection control. These criteria follow consistently with what has been stated in the desired outcomes and nursing prescriptions. What this category concerns is the implementation of actions prescribed in order to achieve the stated desired outcomes. The actions must involve the patient and family, as must all the nursing care plan. The actions are consistent with the nursing prescriptions, in that they carry out into action what has been prescribed. As is all the nursing care plan, the actions are based on currrent scientific knowledge. Just as the plan of care is individualized, so are the actions taken to implement the plan of care.

Including principles of safety in the nursing actions means implementing actions to ensure that the patient is both mentally and physically secure and free from harm or injury. Including principles of infection control means that all actions taken prevent the spread of infection or cross-contamination and incorporate aseptic technique. All six of the above-listed criteria comprise what is expected in the implementation of nursing actions. Once actions are implemented, they are documented in the nurses' notes. Only when nursing prescriptions are formulated and the actions implemented, as defined in the criteria under Standard III, is the plan of care properly implemented.

Standard IV
The fourth and last standard concerns evaluation. It is stated as: "Outcomes of nursing actions are evaluated for further assessment and planning." Once the patient is assessed, the care is planned and implemented into action; then the

outcomes of these actions are evaluated and documented in the nurses' notes. The evaluation of outcomes reflects the effectiveness of the actions and the achievement of the desired outcomes. Evaluation of outcomes and reassessment and planning occur in a sequence of steps that are delineated by the criteria:

1. Data are collected concerning the patient's health status. After nursing actions are implemented, assessment data concerning the patient's health status are collected.
2. These data are compared to the stated desired outcomes.
3. The patient and nurse evaluate whether or not the desired outcome has been achieved.

If the desired outcome has been achieved, the problem may be resolved or simply monitored. Then the problem of next priority may be approached, or from continual assessment, new problems identified. If the desired outcome was not achieved, then a reassessment of the nursing care plan is in order.[8]

Evaluation of the outcome of nursing actions will direct the need to reassess the identified patient problems. Was the problem appropriately assessed and in correct priority? Does the patient really have this problem or is it something else? A reassessment must begin at the assessment and problem identification stage. If all is in order here, the desired outcomes must be reassessed. Is the desired outcome appropriate, realistic, and in correct priority? Is it mutually agreed upon by the patient/family, specific and measureable? Is it individualized and consistent with other health care providers' expectations? Following a thorough assessment of the desired outcome, the nursing prescriptions are reassessed. Are the nursing prescriptions effective in directing actions to be implemented for goal achievement? Are the prescriptions appropriate, realistic, and stated accurately? If outcomes are not achieved, it could be that the prescriptions and resulting nursing actions could be revised without changing the entire care plan. This is an ongoing process, where the nurse tries a variety of nursing actions in an attempt to achieve a desired outcome. Sometimes what works on one patient is not found to work on another. But after evaluating the outcome and reassessing and revising the prescriptions and nursing actions, the desired outcome can be achieved.

The reassessment determines the need for further planning. From the reassessment, new (or revised) patient present/potential problems are determined. The reassessent is continuous and ongoing, even with goal achievement. For example, when desired outcomes are not achieved, the plan of care is reassessed, and revisions are made in order to achieve the desired outcomes. But when problems are resolved or when the patient's status changes (i.e., from preop to postoperative stage), reassessment will direct further care planning and revisions. So the process is continuous and constantly evaluated along the way. Evaluation does not have to occur only as an end stage but should occur throughout the entire process, just as assessment does.[8]

When new or revised patient problems are determined, the rest of the care plan follows, as is defined throughout the standards. The correlated desired outcome is formulated (or revised) consistent with the new patient problem. If a problem's priority is revised, so is the priority of the resulting desired outcome. Revised desired outcomes direct the revised nursing prescriptions and the implementation of revised nursing actions. The evaluation of each step occurs continually, as is stated above. Desired outcomes are continually evaluated for achievement, and the plan of care is continually reassessed, evaluated, and appropriately revised according to changes in the patient's health status.

CONCLUSION

It can be seen from the previous discussion and presentation that the standards are constructed in such a way as to mainly evaluate the process of nursing care. Even Standard IV, concerning evaluation, discusses the "process" of evaluation and the steps to be taken in evaluation. It does not measure patient outcomes according to specific criteria. But the standards presented define the excellence desired in patient care and serve as the structure from which the job descriptions and performance evaluations are developed. The standards are the input into the system and provide one means by which nursing care may be evaluated.

REFERENCES

1. Zimmer, M. J.: Quality assurance for outcomes of patient care. Nursing Clinics of North America, June 1974, 9(3), pp. 305–315.
2. Schmadl, J. C.: Quality assurance: Examination of the concept. Nursing Outlook, July 1979, (27), pp. 462–465.
3. Slee, V. N.: How to know if you have quality control. Hospital Progress, 1972, 53(1), pp. 38–43.
4. Glenin, C.: Formalities of standards of nursing practice using a nursing model. In Conceptual models for nursing practice, J. P. Riehl and C. Roy, New York: Appleton-Century-Crofts, 1974, pp. 234–235.
5. Donabedian, A.: Some issues in evaluating the quality of nursing care. AMJ Public Health, 1969, 59(1), p. 1833.
6. Stevans, B. J.: The nurse as executive. Wakefield, Mass.: Nursing Resources, Inc., 1980, pp. 257–301.
7. Hilger, E. E.: Developing nursing outcome criteria. Nursing Clinics of North America, June 1974, 9(2), pp. 323–330.
8. Yura, H., and Walsh, M.: The nursing process: Assessing, planning, implementing, evaluating (2nd ed.). New York: Appleton-Century-Crofts, 1973, pp. 19–26.
9. American Nurses' Association: Standards of medical-surgical nursing practice. Kansas City, Mo.: ANA, 1974.
10. American Nurses' Association: Standards of nursing practice. Kansas City, Mo.: ANA, 1973.

11. Sherman, J., and Fields, S.: Guide to patient evaluation. Flushing, N. Y.: Medical Examination Publishing Company, Inc., 1974, pp. 26–32.

12. Dugas, B. W.: Introduction to patient care. Philadelphia: W. B. Saunders Company, 1972, pp. 30–31.

13. Brunner, L. S.: The Lippincott manual of nursing practice. Philadelphia: J. B. Lippincott Company, 1974, p. 23.

14. Redman, B. K.: The process of patient teaching in nursing (2nd ed.). St. Louis: C. V. Mosby, 1972, pp. 1–87.

15. Bates, B.: A guide to physical examination. Philadelphia: J. B. Lippincott Company, 1974, p. 5.

BIBLIOGRAPHY

Berg, H. V.: Nursing audit and outcome criteria. Nursing Clinics of North America. June 1974, 9(2).

Cantor, M.: Achieving nursing care standards: Internal and external. Wakefield, Mass.: Nursing Resources, Inc., 1978.

Decka, F., Stevens, L., Vancini, M., amd Wedelzing, L.: Using patient outcome to evaluate community health nursing. Nursing Outlook, 27, April 1979.

Donabedian, A.: Criteria, norms and standards of quality: What do they mean? AMJ Public Health, April 1981, 71, pp. 409–12.

Gallant, B. W., and McLane, A. M.: Outcome criteria: A process for validation at the unit level. JONA, Jan. 1979, (9), pp. 14–21.

Inzer, F., and Aspinwall, M. J.: Evaluating patient outcomes. Nursing Outlook, 29, March 1981, pp. 178–181.

Martin, E. J., Finneran, M. R.,: A teaching design: Standards of practice as a liaison for peer review. Perspect Psychiatric Care, November/December 1980, (18), pp. 242–8.

Stevens, B. J.: ANA's standards for nursing services: How do they measure up? JONA, May 1976, (6), pp. 29–31.

Taylor, J. W.: Measuring the outcomes of nursing care. Nursing Clinics of North America, June 1974, 9(2), pp. 337–348.

Zimmer, M. J., and Associates: Guidelines for development of outcome criteria. Nursing Clinics of North America, June 1974, 9(2), pp. 317–320.

3

Job Descriptions

A job description is exactly what it says—it describes the job. It is written statements that list the expected behavior of an employee. Despite this definition, many job descriptions consist of vague and ambiguous statements, with no clear explanation of what is expected. Some job descriptions are completely separate from the standards of practice, defining job behavior with no indication of the expectations defined in the standards. Other job descriptions have no connection to the employee's evaluation form. So the employee is told what is expected and evaluated on another set of general principles unrelated to the job description.[1] The purpose of this chapter is to define job descriptions, discuss their essential components, demonstrate examples of statements in a specific job description, and discuss their importance in the overall organizational system.

A DEFINITION

For our purposes, a job description is a set of statements, based upon standards of practice, that comprises the employee's contract with the institution. As a contract, it serves as a base for the performance evaluation, which in turn ensures compliance with the contract. What this means is, first, the job description is an incorporation of the standards of nursing practice. As described in the introduction, it is the second component of the system and derives input from the standards. If assessment of the patient's health status is a nursing standard, this statement is written into the job description as "Assesses the health status of assigned patients on the unit as outlined in the nursing standards," or something to that effect. Specific criteria under the standard can be added to provide the detailed expectation of performance.

The second part of the definition concerns the employee's contract with the institution. When a new employee comes to an institution, the first thing that should be discussed and agreed upon is the job description. In fact, it is important for an employee who is "just looking" to have a copy of a job description so that she will know from the beginning what the job entails, what her responsibilities are, and what is expected from her.* The decision to hire new employees should be contingent upon their reading, understanding, and agreeing to the requirements defined in the job description.[2] This agreement should be documented at the end of the description with their signature under a statement such as, "I have read and understand the above job description. I am accepting the responsibilities and agree to fulfill these and other duties as assigned." (See Fig. 3-1.) This seals the contract and both parties are aware of the expected behaviors.

The last statement in the contract concerning "Other duties as assigned" is necessary to allow for unspecific responsibilities. There is no way a job description can list absolutely every duty an employee will ever need to perform. For example, if a nursing assistant is at the nurses' station, she cannot refuse to take a requisition slip to the laboratory simply because it was not defined in her job description. This is a safety measure necessary to the institution.

The third part of the definition of a job description is that it serves as the format for the performance evaluation, which, in turn, monitors the upholding of the contract. The job description states the standards in operational terms, in order for them to be implemented. These statements are then used to comprise the performance evaluation. This transformation from the standards through to the performance evaluation is the thruput stage. Every item specified as a job requirement becomes an evaluation item on the performance evaluation. (Refer to the job descriptions and performance evaluations in Chapters 7 through 13.) If the employee receives a satisfactory rating on the evaluation, she is upholding her contract to fulfill the duties on the job description. (See Chapter 4 for more information concerning the performance evaluation.)

Another important reason why the job description is a base for the performance evaluation is that the employee is evaluated on exactly what is required of her. The employee knows what is expected and is evaluated on that expected behavior. This makes the job description more meaningful and valid. The job description should never stand alone but should only exist as an extension of the standards and as a component in the evaluation process.

STATEMENT OF UNDERSTANDING AND ACCEPTANCE
I have read and understand the above job description. I am accepting the responsibilities and agree to fulfill these and other duties as assigned.

_____   _____
Employee's Signature   Date

Figure 3-1 Standard form for understanding and acceptance of job description.

*For simplicity, throughout this book a nurse will be referred to using *she* or *her* and the patient as *he* or *him*. The authors hope that no offense is taken by the reader.

ELEMENTS OF THE JOB DESCRIPTION

The job description consists of other important elements, other than the nursing standards. These elements may be more specific in a job with less responsibility, such as a task-oriented job. With jobs having higher levels of responsibility, the employee may perform various skills and duties in order to achieve the job expectations. Therefore, more freedom is allowed in carrying out the job when every detail is not specified.[1]

Some important elements in the job descriptions are title, position requirements, accountability, and position summary.[3] The title simply states for whom the job description is written. Requirements for the job may be divided into position requirements and professional requirements.

Position requirements state what is required in order to be hired to fill the position. It will depend on the level of responsibility, as well as availability of personnel. For instance, the job of director of nursing service would call for a registered nurse with a certain amount of experience. Depending on the institution, experience may be required in clinical practice, nursing administration, as well as in research and consulting. Requirements such as experience and educational background will depend on JCAH recommendations, such as a baccalaureate degree being preferred and availability of higher educated nurses. In an area where a baccalaureate degreed nurse is hard to find, it would be unrealistic to require a master's degree in nursing for this position. (It may just state "preferred.") But in a large teaching institute, it might not be unrealistic to require a doctorate degree along with evidence of publishing, as well as clinical experience in administration. The position requirements on the job descriptions will reflect the needs of the institution, as well as its philosophy and available resource persons.

Professional requirements refer to what is required by the person as a professional. It could be guidelines recommended by the nurses' association or the philosophy and decision of the nursing service. These requirements include personal growth, activities in the nursing profession, continuing education and certification, involvement in community activities, and other professional involvements. They may be required on some job descriptions, or recommended on others, and used as a determining factor for hiring purposes. Mandatory requirements, as established by the nurses' association (such as mandatory continuing education), would not be considered under this section.

Job descriptions need to define the lines of accountability. It may be taken for granted that a nurse is accountable for all behaviors listed in her job description, but the description should be written to clarify this point. To whom the nurse is accountable refers to what person she answers. A job description might state that a nursing supervisor is accountable to the Director of Nursing Service, the patient, and the family. This reflects the organizational chart of the institution as well as the philosophy of the nursing service. But it should be clear to whom, and for what, the employee is accountable.

A position summary is a few statements or a paragraph describing briefly the main functions and responsibilities of the position. It is usually general and gives the employee an overview of the job description.[2]

LIST OF DUTIES

Following the summary is a list of duties, responsibilities, and tasks. These should vary, depending on the level of responsibility, and clearly delineate differences of responsibility between different positions.

In referring to the Medical-Surgical Registered Nurse job description in Chapter 7, it can be seen that the duties/responsibilities are divided into four sections. These sections are assessment, planning, implementation, and evaluation; they divide the related responsibilities accordingly. For example, the registered nurse's responsibility in identifying problems on the unit and assessing any need for improvement would go under the assessment category. Also, the job requirements related to the assessment Standard I would be categorized under assessment. It can also be seen that all the criteria for each standard is listed to further explain what is expected behavior for the nurse concerning assessment, planning, implementation, and evaluation.

The statements in the nurse's job description should reflect not only the requirements of the nursing service but the philosophy of the nurses themselves.[4] Each year a committee of nurse representatives gets together to review the job descriptions and revise them according to their beliefs and the needs of the hospital. For example, the nurses felt that setting self-objectives, working toward those objectives, and evaluating achievement of the objectives was important. They wanted this included in their job descriptions and in their evaluations. They also felt that problem identification and involvement with changes on the unit were essential to quality nursing care. It was the consensus of the nursing staff that these things be included in the job descriptions.

Certain items on the job description can be misleading and ambiguous and difficult to measure. "Demonstrating clinical competency at all times" is one of these. How do you measure clinical competency? What specific criteria are used? This becomes a complicated and confusing process, and one that needs to be addressed if the nursing service decides to list it in the job description. The nurses on this committee decided that by properly implementing all items on the job description a nurse would be demonstrating competency. It is important that all items are evaluated to make sure they are clearly stated and measurable. This is essential for performance evaluation purposes.

Another item that is hard to define is "Displays a good attitude at all times." How do you measure a good attitude? The nurses felt that attitude was so important that it should be integrated into all aspects of the job. So they decided to integrate attitude as a determining criterion when evaluating performance. In other words, the difference between satisfactory and above-average performance could sometimes be determined by attitude. They felt that only one item related to attitude was not sufficient and was difficult to measure as well. (Refer to the next chapter for further explanation of evaluation.)

UTILIZING THE JOB DESCRIPTION

The job description is actively utilized in the orientation of new nurses.[2] For teaching purposes, it demonstrates the content of the nursing standards and what they, as nurses, must do to achieve the standards. Each phase of the job description can be taken separately, and the necessary skills, knowledge, pertinent policies, and procedures related to that phase can be discussed. For instance, when discussing the assessment phase of the job description, the nursing interview and assessment form and the relating policies concerning patient assessment are also reviewed. The nurse is taken through all procedures related to assessment and shown how the job description is actually carried out into action. Once all four phases are covered, the nurse is well aware of expected behaviors, of the content of the nursing standards, of how she will be evaluated, and of all aspects of the nursing process.

CONCLUSION

Job descriptions relate to patient care, as they define the actions to be taken in the delivery of that care. When reading through the job descriptions in later chapters, many similarities will be observed. This is attributed to the fact that the nursing process is the framework for nursing practice. These processes, involving four continuous, interrelated steps, are the same for patient care in any area.[5] The Maternal-Child Health Nurse will assess, plan, implement, and evaluate her patient care, just as the emergency nurse will do in her area. The processes are broad and cover any area of nursing. The specific responsibilities related to a specialty area make these job descriptions different. By presenting examples of job descriptions in various areas, much time and energy can be saved for the reader in developing her own form.

The point to keep in mind is the integration and interaction of the nursing standards, job descriptions, and performance evaluations. Chapter 4 will assist in conceptualizing this system.

REFERENCES

1. Stevens, B. J.: The nurse as executive (2nd ed.). Wakefield, Mass.: Nursing Resources, Inc., 1980, pp. 304, 68–70.
2. Christopher, W. I.: Management Improvement for Hospitals. St. Louis: W. I. Christopher and Associates, Inc., 1982.
3. Brockenshire, A., and Hattstaldt, M. J.: Revising job descriptions: A consensus approach. Supervisor Nurse, March 1980, pp. 16–20.
4. Ignatavicius, D., and Griffith J.: Job analysis: The basis of effective appraisal. JONA, July/August, 1982, pp. 37–41.
5. Yura, H., and Walsh, M.: The nursing process: Assessing, planning, implementing, evaluating (2nd ed.). New York: Appleton-Century-Crofts, 1973, p. 1.

BIBLIOGRAPHY

Fitton, J.: What health visitors say they do—A job description approach. Health Visit, April 1981, (54), p. 159.

Raniere, T. M., Parker, J. E.: Job description: Key to your future. Occup. Health Nurs, Aug. 1981, (29), pp. 9–11.

Redman, B. K.: The process of patient teaching in nursing. St. Louis: C. V. Mosby Co., 1972, pp. 59–69.

Rinaldi, M.: Updating job descriptions: A useful tool. Nursing Homes, March 1976, p. 14.

Shaw, O., Martyn, R.: Taking C.A.R.E. of employees. Dimens. Health Serv., January 1981, (58), pp. 26–27.

Tescher, B. E., and Colanecchio, R.: Definition of a standard for clinical nursing practice. JONA, March 1977, pp. 32–44.

Umiker, W. U.: Good position descriptions help fit the employee to the job. MLO, September 1981, (13), pp. 32–36.

4

Performance Evaluation

Performance evaluation is the process of evaluating the nurse's (or employee's) performance, using some predetermined guide or form. The development of a usable, valid, and reliable form is a time-consuming task but produces many desirable and positive results. A reliable performance evaluation indicates the nurse's level of achievement of expectations defined in the job descriptions. It can reflect the performance status of various nursing units, as well as that of the overall nursing service. Developed and used effectively, the performance evaluation can serve many purposes that contribute to improvement of the nursing service and delivery of patient care.[1] These and other topics, such as development of a performance evaluation and its initiation into the nursing management system, will be presented in this chapter.

The performance evaluation should be based on defined and agreed-upon job expectations at the time of hiring.[2] It should never be considered as an independent entity, but only as part of the overall nursing system.[3] A good performance evaluation can increase the employee's motivation to improve by providing a reward (such as praise, money, promotion) for positive behaviors. It can identify problems early in an employee's performance, focus on special skills and abilities that need improvement, and guide the employee toward appropriate desired behavior.[4] Developed and implemented properly, the performance evaluation can reflect compliance with nursing standards and the quality of care provided by the nursing staff.

With these points in mind, a committee of nurses set about formulating performance evaluations and helped to effectively initiate them into a nursing system. From their experience, the following guidelines were recommended for writing and introducing new criteria-based performance evaluations.

FORMULATING THE PERFORMANCE EVALUATION

The first and most important requirement is that the performance evaluations be derived directly from the job descriptions. This ensures that the employee's evaluation is being based upon job expectations. The employees must have time to accept new job descriptions before formulating the evaluations. A 3-month waiting period following the inservicing and initiation of the job descriptions is necessary before implementing this tool. It is imperative that all employees are knowledgeable and agree upon the statements in their job descriptions, because this is the exact criteria by which they will be evaluated. During the 3-month period, the job descriptions can be revised as necessary and reinserviced, until finally accepted by the nursing service employees.

Each item on the job description is then transferred verbatim to the performance evaluation form according to the same four categories of assessment, planning, implementation, and evaluation. This way the employee is directly evaluated on the agreed-upon standards of performance, and all items have been previously accepted as sound and creditable by nursing service employees. This also forms a system whereby each of the three components, standards, job descriptions, and performance evaluation, are interrelated. The three components constantly interreact as the performance evaluation evaluates the implementation of the job description, and therefore compliance with the nursing standards.

For example, Standard I of the Standards of Medical-Surgical Nursing Practice states: "Assessment is the identification and gathering of data concerning the health status of the patient. This process is complete, continuous and systematic." Then the criteria for evaluation are listed. On the job description these statements are written as: "Assesses the health status of assigned patients on the unit, as outlined in the nursing standards." Each criterion for evaluation is then listed below this statement. This way the exact required behavior is specified. The RN performance evaluation reads "_____ Assesses the health status of assigned patients on the unit as outlined in the nursing standards." Each criterion is then listed for inclusion in the evaluation process of this item. The results of the evaluation or the rating is written to the left of the item, in the blank space provided.

If the nurse is evaluated as "satisfactory," this reflects satisfactory implementation of the assessment item on the job description and satisfactory compliance with the assessment standard in the standards of nursing practice. An "above average" or "exceptional" rating would relate to a higher-quality nursing assessment. If the performance is evaluated as "unsatisfactory," the job description and nursing standards have not been implemented properly, and corrective action must be taken. These actions will be discussed later in the chapter.

A RATING SCALE

It is important that the performance evaluation objectively measures the employee's performance. A valid and reliable procedure must be developed that is also trusted by the nursing staff. There are different formats from which to choose. For instance, essay forms are more or less a sheet of paper on which the evaluator writes a narrative type of evaluation of the employee. Management by objectives involves evaluating performance against predetermined objectives written by the employee.[3] These forms were not acceptable, as inclusion of job description expectations could not be guaranteed with these types of formats. After a thorough investigation, this committee decided on a rating scale to which various items can be listed, and the evaluator can rate the employee's performance according to an established scale.[3] This scale is divided into four categories: Unsatisfactory, or does not meet job requirements; Satisfactory, or meets job requirements; Above Average, or exceeds job requirements; and Exceptional, or displays outstanding performance.

A MEASUREMENT TOOL FOR EVALUATION

After the components of the performance evaluation are written from the job description, and the rating scale is determined, the procedure for evaluation has to be delineated. In order for an employee to be rated, the categories *unsatisfactory, satisfactory, above average,* and *exceptional performance* should be defined.[1] A measurement tool is necessary to serve as a guide and to provide rationale for decision making in evaluating the employee's performance.[5]

This tool may be developed over several weeks with participation from supervisors, the nursing committee, and discussion at staff meetings. The Medical-Surgical RN Performance Evaluation can be used for developing the original tool, and the various nursing specialties and LPN evaluation tools can be developed from this. An example of an RN tool is presented at the end of the chapter in the section entitled "Medical-Surgical Registered Nurse, Criteria for Performance Evaluation." Presented there is each item on the form, with the agreed-upon definition of the four ratings. These definitions should be made available to nursing staff members, and they must be aware of the procedure for determining their ranking on all items on the performance evaluation. When the staff participates in the tool's development, they will believe the definitions to be fair and accurate.

VALIDITY AND RELIABILITY

After the development of the performance evaluation form and the tool for evaluating each item, the procedure should be tested for validity and reliability. Validity means the form measures the performance of the employee as defined in the job description.[4] This can be tested in the following way: The committee evaluates various members of the nursing staff using the new form. Then, using the job description as a guide, two of the supervisors collect data on the Kardex, the care plans, the nurses' notes, and other chart forms and observe the nurses providing care and interviewing the patients. They compare the data concerning these nurses' performance with the committee's evaluations to determine if the nurses are actually doing what the evaluation forms indicate. If the results are congruent, one can be satisfied that the form is valid. If the results are not congruent, the problem areas must be identified and corrected. Then the procedure is repeated. At this time items can be evaluated to determine that they are measurable. Revisions may have to be made in certain items so that they are objectively worded and measurable to facilitate their validity and reliability. In addition, because the evaluation form is identical to the job description, it automatically evaluates the required job expectations. This contributes to its validity.

Reliability concerns the results of an evaluation being the same, even when performed by different supervisors.[4] In other words, all employees must be evaluated in the same objective manner and obtain the same score, no matter which supervisor is evaluating them. Before this can be tested, the management personnel must be thoroughly inserviced on the performance evaluation procedure. The procedure should be clearly written step by step, indicating who does the evaluating for which employee. (See Appendix 4-1.) The scoring procedure must also be written so that each supervisor can practice and be comfortable in tabulating the scores of the evaluations. (See Appendix 4-2.)

The management personnel can be inserviced in a concentrated 3-week period. Each day for 1 hour different aspects of performance evaluation can be discussed. Principles of interviewing, data collection, objectivity, feedback mechanisms and correction of deficient behaviors, and recommendations for improvement in performance are some of the many issues requiring discussion throughout this period. By the end of the 3 weeks, the nursing management should understand what is expected of them and be thoroughly versed in all aspects of the various performance evaluations. The management should also be in agreement regarding the definition of the rating for each item. It should be decided during this time that, when an employee's performance is borderline or unusually difficult to assess, two of the supervisors or head nurses who work with this employee get together and complete the evaluation as a joint effort. This would assist in remaining objective and providing more feedback for the employee.

Following this inservice, the managers should test the forms for reliability. A head nurse and supervisor on the same unit can evaluate an employee separately and then get together on the results. If any of the ratings differ, they are discussed and the managers come to agreement on the rating. This should be done at least three times by all managers until the results are the same within an agreed-upon number. Throughout the initiation of these forms, the Director of Nursing, or other appropriate persons, should closely monitor the evaluations. During this time each manager should obtain a second opinion in order to further verify and substantiate the ratings and ensure objectivity and correctness. After a period of 6 months, when both management and staff are comfortable with this procedure, this is not required on every evaluation.

PERFORMANCE EVALUATION SCORES

After the implementation of the performance evaluation system, the results of the scoring can be used in several ways. First of all, and the most obvious, it serves as a reward for the employee. By working hard to improve and seeing this work noticed and written on the evaluation, the employee feels recognition for her efforts.[4] Often policies contribute to this reward, such as a policy stating that promotion is based upon the performance evaluation score. Monetary rewards may be related to the performance evaluation, such as the merit raise system presented in Chapter 5. All these things help to reward the employee for good work and to promote improvement and motivation to continue the effort.[6]

The performance evaluation scores can also reflect problem areas, strengths and weaknesses, not only in an individual score but in group scores. By adding the total scores for each item in the RN's evaluation on a specific unit, information about the RNs on the unit can be identified.[1] If all RNs in a unit are "excellent" on patient assessment, they may be involved in the teaching of nurses on other units. Or if, in the area on planning for home health care some nurses are evaluated "S" but are consistently documented with comments recommending improvement, an inservice may be needed for these nurses. By scanning the totals of the evaluations, strengths and weaknesses can be identified for all nursing staff members and used in needs analysis, planning, and reevaluation of the system.

The evaluation defines areas in need of improvement, not only by the scores but by the examples and recommendations written in the comment section under each item and on the back scoring page. These comments supply the employees with specific areas to work toward and helps them to develop self-objectives. By rewarding good behavior and citing ways to improve in other areas, the employee is likely to want to continue to improve. Once rewarded, the chance of continual positive feedback, increased monetary gain, and personal recognition can serve as a motivator.[7]

CORRECTION OF DEFICIENT BEHAVIOR

The performance evaluation must have policies and procedures to enforce the correcting of deficient behavior or noncompliance with the standards. Without corrective actions, the unsatisfactory scores would never be improved, and the system would have no feedback mechanism.

The results of the individual and group performance evaluations feed back into the system. The Supervisors, Head Nurses, and Director of Nurses evaluate the scores. "Satisfactory" is considered the minimal level for compliance with the standards. The individuals may be given special classes and assistance in ways to improve, but these scores are acceptable. The system can remain in operation. "Above average" and "excellent" scores serve as feedback concerning a higher level of performance. It shows which areas are strongest and where the nursing service excels. An unsatisfactory score does not permit the system to operate. This feedback is identified by the immediate supervisor, and policies dictate certain steps to be taken.

For example, an employee should not be allowed to have an unsatisfactory score on an item twice in a row. This prevents the continuation of unsatisfactory behavior in the same area and impels the employee to improve any deficient performance. (See Appendix 4-1.) Employees should be placed on probation when receiving unsatisfactory as a total score, and certain penalties must be enforced. Policies should be written to lead to the dismissal of employees who consistently score below satisfactory. Counseling, special inservices, and prolonged orientation or reorientation procedures may be in order. But many efforts must be taken to assist the employee to improve. If no improvement is evidenced, the employee must be dismissed, and, therefore, the deficiency does not remain in the system. There should be no exceptions for these rules, or the standards will fail to be achieved. Every effort must be taken to correct unsatisfactory behavior and to improve satisfactory behavior. Also, the comments and recommendations written throughout and at the end of the evaluation are a type of corrective action. These remarks are used in the employee's development of self-objectives and are referred to at the next interview session. The evaluator expects to see improvement in these areas and uses them for consideration in decision making.

OBJECTIVITY

In order for performance evaluation results to reflect compliance with nursing standards, they must be objective. Objectivity is monitored in various ways, some of which have been discussed. By participating with staff in gathering information and consulting with other management people in completing the evaluation, objectivity is facilitated. Also, by requiring specific documentation of examples of any unsatisfactory or exceptional scores, the supervisor must be objective in marking these scores. The management people must be inserviced thoroughly and continually concerning objectivity and accurate data collection. They must become proficient at gathering information concerning their personnel and possess the documentation to substantiate their decisions. Also, it is wise to provide a formal time for evaluation other than the annual time so that employees are well aware of their status and areas in need of improvement.[6] The whole idea is to provide feedback and to help the employee achieve the highest scores possible. This way the employee is rewarded, the standards are achieved, and the hospital benefits.

The Director of Nursing should continually monitor the supervisor's and head nurse's evaluations and ensure that they are well documented. She should also have spot checks performed by management personnel from other units to see if, in reality, these employees are doing what the evaluations reflect. This is a good way to monitor the system as well as to determine compliance with nursing standards.

For example, all nurses are required to initial the care plans they write on the Kardexes. An evaluation may be turned in on a nurse that is rated as exceptional. The supervisor may check the Kardex and look for evidence of the criteria listed under the excellent rating for "planning." She can determine if all criteria are present, and at the same time determine whether the planning standard is being met. These spot checks should be performed on various units on a monthly basis.

EVALUATION

The evaluation forms should be formally evaluated at least annually. In addition, if consistently low scores are being produced by the staff, both the evaluating process and the components of the system need to be reevaluated; for instance, the supervisors may not be providing appropriate feedback and opportunity for improvement, or the nurses may be unsure of their job expectations. Staff meetings or reinservicing may be necessary. Whenever low scores are evidenced, the reason should be identified and discussed by management and the appropriate corrective action taken. It may even occur that certain elements in the standards need changing or revision or that the job descriptions don't clearly state the expectations. So the scores and the annual evaluation of the performance evaluation forms may serve as feedback for revisions in other components of the system. Whenever a revision is made in one area of a component, such as the performance evaluation, the other components, standards, and job descriptions must also be revised.

CONCLUSION

Performance Evaluation, in contrast to the evaluation phase of the nursing process, helps to evaluate the process of nursing care delivery rather than the patient outcomes. This system focuses on "process." The scores of the evaluations, when combined with other quality assurance activities and mechanisms to correct deficiencies, can assure that quality care is provided.[8] Together with other evaluation activities, the performance evaluation can serve as a valid indicator of compliance with nursing standards. The three components, standards, job descriptions, and performance evaluations, fit together in a system to maintain standards of nursing practice. It is one part, or a subsystem, in the overall system of quality control.

MEDICAL-SURGICAL REGISTERED NURSE: CRITERIA FOR PERFORMANCE EVALUATION

The following is a tool for completing the Registered Nurse Performance Evaluation Form. This is not intended as a comprehensive guide, but to provide examples to which to refer when completing the performance evaluation. (See Medical-Surgical RN Performance Evaluation, Chapter 7.)

Assessment

1. Assesses the number and level of personnel needed to provide quality patient care on the unit and collaborates with the Head Nurse or Supervisor in adjusting staffing and assignment.

Explanation

Following report, the Registered Nurse assesses the number and expertise of the personnel and compares this with the patient classification to ensure that quality care can be delivered according to patient's needs. She assesses the assignments to see that they are fair, based on the patient's needs and personnel's qualifications. According to her assessment, the Registered Nurse makes adjustments in assignments, requests more help, or collaborates with Supervisor or Head Nurse on schedule changes for the next shift (or next day). This assessment is also a basis for deciding whether personnel can be sent to another hall or unit.

Evaluation Guide

U – Considers only the number of patients—not the classification. "Never has enough help." Uncooperative in making changes in assignments or staffing. Rarely adjusts assignments, even with changes in census or patient acuity. Cannot give rationale to substantiate the need, when requesting additional staff.

S – Is aware of patient classification and needs, staff expertise, and ability to care for the patients. Substantiates reasons for requesting more help. Adjusts assignments based on the above rationale. Can determine whether number and level of personnel available are equivalent to the patient care required. Can determine whether assignments are appropriate. Is cooperative in accepting changes in staffing, or assignments, when requested by Supervisor and Head Nurse—based on patient classification and sound rationale.

A – Performs all behaviors described in S. Continually assesses changes in census and patient acuity and adjusts assignments and delegation of duties accordingly throughout the shift.

E – Performs all behaviors in A. Assesses the staffing needs of the on-coming shift and collaborates with Head Nurse or Supervisor and can provide rationale for changes needed, according to this assessment. Considers the needs of the other units, as well as her own unit and includes this concern in decisions for staffing and assignment changes. Includes assessment rationale in suggesting changes or adjustments in the next day's staffing and assignments.

2. Assesses the delivery of nursing care on the unit and identifies problems and any need for improvement.

Explanation
  The Registered Nurse constantly observes the delivery of nursing care
  and the performance of the personnel providing that care. The Registered Nurse makes rounds and assesses the patients to see that appropriate care is being delivered in order to meet their needs. From this
  assessment, the Registered Nurse identifies any problems that may be
  occurring on the unit, among personnel, etc. The Registered Nurse
  identifies areas needing improvement, or management of personnel
  concerning skills and knowledge, materials, or resources needed.

Evaluation Guide
U – Never or rarely identifies needs on the unit. Goes without equipment
  or forms needed without verbalizing the deficiency. May verbalize
  problems and needs but rarely has rationale on which to base the
  problems.
S – When asked, will identify needs and problems on the unit. Gives
  rationale for these problems, from assessment.
A – Is self-motivated to communicate assessment and identification of
  needs and problems to supervisory personnel. Identifies needs concerning additional knowledge and skills that would improve the delivery of care, based on sound rationale.
E – Performs all behaviors described in A. Identifies potential needs and
  problems and communicates these to supervisory personnel.

3. Assesses the health status of assigned patients on the unit as outlined in
   the nursing standards.
   3.1 Completes a comprehensive patient history and physical, including
       patient interview, psychological and physical assessment, as well as
       patient's perception of illness.
   3.2 Collects data initially and on a continual basis from the patient,
       family, and significant others, health care providers, individuals,
       and/or agencies in the community.
   3.3 Collects data by interview, observation, inspection, auscultation,
       palpation, and reports and records.
   3.4 Organizes assessment data so that they are accurate, complete, ac-
       cessible, and that they remain confidential.
   3.5 Communicates assessment data in an orderly fashion by recording,
       updating, and communicating among the health team daily and
       revising as appropriate.

Evaluation Guide
U – Fails to meet criteria listed under assessment (3.1–3.5).
S – Satisfies all criteria (3.1–3.5) and completes initial assessment note
  within 30 minutes.
A – Performs all behaviors described in S. Completes assessment forms
  from previous shifts and adds pertinent information from her assessment. Seeks out additional information from all possible sources for
  the patient assessment. Communicates the patient's problems and care
  plan to the oncoming shift.
E – Performs all behaviors described in A. Assesses slight alterations in
  the patient's health status and documents these changes.

Planning

1. Serves on hospital committees and helps to review and revise policies and procedures as directed by Head Nurse or Supervisor.

Explanation

The Registered Nurse as a professional participates in nursing service committees (such as Quality Assurance or Policy and Procedure committee).

Evaluation Guide

U – Never or rarely serves on committees, even when requested.

S – Serves on committees, when requested.

A – Volunteers to serve on committees, contributes, and actively participates.

E – Volunteers to serve on committees, contributes, and actively participates. Demonstrates evidence of committee work on the unit. Includes information obtained from committee work in documentation, interactions, and direct patient care.

2. Plans and develops self-objectives.

Explanation

The Registered Nurse assesses her own skills, knowledge, and interactions and identifies personal objectives. These objectives are goals to work toward and are intended to improve her overall performance, as well as enhance her professional growth and knowledge.

Evaluation Guide

U – Does not identify self-objectives from the performance evaluation.

S – Plans and develops self-objectives and documents this on the annual evaluation. Sets target dates for completion.

A – Develops self-objectives from not only the performance evaluation but from personal experiences and assessments as well. When developing objectives, sets priorities and identifies resources needed and areas of delegation. Documents this on the performance evaluation form.

E – Performs all behaviors described in A. Maintains a personal list of self-objectives, and from the self-assessment adds new objectives every 3 months.

3. Plans ways to solve problems and to make improvements on the unit, in collaboration with supervisory personnel.

Explanation

From assessment of the delivery of nursing care, the Registered Nurse plans ways to solve identified problems or to prevent potential problems. The Registered Nurse should participate in planning ways to improve the care given on her unit. For example, if patients that are NPO are repeatedly being fed in the mornings, the Registered Nurse identifies this as a problem. Next, she futher assesses reasons and causes for these occurrences. If she identifies the problem as the personnel not checking the NPO list and trays before serving them, or that the NPO signs are not being read on the patient's door before serving the tray, the Registered Nurse would try to resolve this problem. One way is to participate in the unit meeting and discuss the correct procedure with personnel. The Registered Nurse may participate in planning the unit meeting and developing a better procedure for checking the trays.

Evaluation Guide

U – Never participates in planning ways to improve the activities on the unit.

S – When asked, will participate in planning ways to solve problems and make improvements on the unit. Attends 90% of unit and staff meetings to discuss needs and problems relating to patient care.

A – Is self-motivated to communicate ideas and actively suggests solutions for problems and ways to improve activities on the unit. Attends 90% of unit and staff meetings.

E – From assessment, identifies potential problems and plans ways to prevent these problems. Considers long-range improvements in the delivery of nursing care on the unit. Communicates this information to supervisory personnel. Attends 90% of unit and staff meetings.

4. Completes a written care plan for assigned patients on the unit.
   4.1 Identifies the patient's present/potential problems from the patient assessment: (a) patient's health status is determined; (b) health status is compared to the norms; and (c) problems are given priority according to impact upon the patient's health status.
   4.2 Formulates desired outcomes, specific to the patient problems and established norms.
   4.3 Ensures that desired outcomes are mutually agreed upon by the patient and nurse and are: (a) specific; (b) measurable within a certain time frame; and (c) consistent with other health provider's expectations.
   4.4 Incorporates home health care into the patient's desired outcomes. This includes but is not limited to teaching about the disease process and complications, medications, diet, exercise/activity, self-care techniques, and materials and available support systems and resources.

Explanation

Plans the care for assigned patients, as outlined by the criteria, and directs others in the planning of the patient's care.

Evaluation Guide

U – Fails to meet the criteria outlined under care planning.

S – Satisfies all criteria listed under care planning and documents it within a 24-hour period.

A – Following the initial assessment, formulates and documents the identified patient problems and desired outcomes on all new admissions during the 8-hour shift.

E – Performs all behaviors described in A. From continual assessment, updates the problem list and desired outcomes for previous shifts on all assigned patients each day.

Implementation

    1. Implements activities necessary to meeting self-objectives.

Explanation

    The Registered Nurse implements activities necessary to achieve the self-objectives developed and documented.

U – Does not implement activities to achieve self-objectives.

S – With assistance from the Supervisor, implements activities necessary to achieve self-objectives.

A – Is self-motivated to initiate actions to achieve self-objectives. If unsuccessful, implements other actions.

E – Is creative and utilizes resources and input from personnel in implementing activities necessary to achieve self-objectives.

    2. Participates in implementing planned change and activities to improve nursing service.

Explanation

    The Registered Nurse participates in planned changes, such as initiating new forms or implementing new policies and procedures. She is supportive of changes and understands the rationale for the changes.

Evaluation Guide

U – Is uncooperative in implementing planned change.

S – With encouragement from supervisory personnel, will participate in activities to improve nursing service.

A – Volunteers and is enthusiastic about implementing planned change and activities to improve nursing service. Actively participates.

E – Performs all behaviors described in A. Encourages others to participate in activities to improve nursing service. Is dedicated to making it work.

    3. Holds self accountable for the delivery of quality nursing care.

Explanation

    The Registered Nurse can justify and explain her actions. She holds herself answerable for all activities related to care of assigned patient.

Evaluation Guide

U – Never or rarely takes responsibility for the care given to assigned patients. Always offers excuses or reasons for not being aware of activities relating to patient care.

S – Can explain all nursing actions and is aware of the effect of actions on patient care.

A – Can explain and takes responsibility for care given by self and personnel under authority, such as LPNs, aides, and orderlies.

E – Values self-accountability highly. Directs others' actions and requests information pertinent to patient care. Considers self as being integral to the patient's care and when on duty feels responsible for any activities concerning assigned patients, including procedures performed in other departments.

4. Promotes harmonious relationships and favorable attitudes among the health care team.

Explanation

The Registered Nurse cooperates with other members of the health care team and does not allow personal differences to interfere with patient care. She sets an example for other employees by demonstrating a positive attitude about everyone "working together" for the betterment of the patient. The Registered Nurse minimizes interpersonal conflicts and attempts to cooperate with others.

Evaluation Guide

U – Exaggerates personal differences, is uncooperative about working with certain persons, displays a negative attitude when presented with changes.

S – With encouragement from supervisory personnel, accepts changes and forgets personal differences and attempts to "get along" with all members of the health care team.

A – Is self-motivated to improve and maintain a good attitude and harmonious relations among other personnel and members of the health care team.

E – Promotes positive relations and attitudes among personnel and acts as a role model by displaying enthusiasm and motivation for harmony among health care team.

5. Supports and adheres to administrative and nursing service policies and procedures.

Explanation

Is knowledgeable of and complies with policies and procedures.

Evaluation Guide

U – Rarely is knowledgeable of policies or procedures affecting the Registered Nurse's practice and often does not comply with policies and procedures.

S – Is knowledgeable of and complies with policies and procedures affecting nursing. When requested, assists with review and revision of policies and procedures.

A – Performs all behaviors described in S. Refers to policy and procedure book to verify actions or answer questions by other staff members. Reviews the books periodically to maintain familiarity with policies and procedures.

E – Performs all behaviors described in A. Always complies with policies and procedures. If does not, communicates the rationale for noncompliance to the supervisor and/or recommends revision in the policy or procedure.

6. Assists with the orientation of new employees.

Explanation

The Registered Nurse works as a preceptor with a new Registered Nurse on a day-to-day basis, according to the orientation procedure. The Registered Nurse assists with the orientation of LPNs, Nursing Assistants, and Unit Secretaries.

Evaluation Guide

U – Refuses or is uncooperative in serving as a preceptor for a new employee. If accepts, will not work closely with the new Registered Nurse and leaves the new nurse to learn on her own.

S – When asked, accepts the role as preceptor. Follows the orientation procedure and works closely with the new nurse by demonstrating skills and allowing the nurse to slowly gain responsibility after showing competence to do so.

A – Performs all behaviors described in S. Requests to serve as preceptor. Is enthusiastic about helping new LPNs, NAs, Orderlies, and Unit Secretaries and goes out of way to be helpful. Works closely with the Inservice Director in providing orientation.

E – Performs all behaviors described in A. Makes new employees feel at home. Reviews and explains policies and procedure with which the employee is unfamiliar. Seeks out learning experiences that would be beneficial to the employee and is well aware of her learning needs.

7. Acts rapidly and effectively and manages self, patients, and other employees during any emergency situation.

Explanation

The Registered Nurse is knowledgeable of policies, procedures, and equipment needed during emergencies. She remains calm and effectively manages self and all people involved in the emergency.

Evaluation Guide

U – Is not familiar with emergency procedures or equipment and tends to lose control during emergencies.

S – Follows policies and procedures during emergencies. Remains calm and maintains control. Is familiar with emergency equipment.

A – Performs all behaviors described in S. Manages and directs LPNs, Nursing Assistants, Orderlies, and patients/families during emergencies.

E – Performs all behaviors described in A. Provides a calming effect for other personnel. Provides emotional support for families and patients when appropriate. Takes charge until the appropriate persons arrive on the scene.

8. Attends required inservice education programs.

Evaluation Guide

U – Does not attend all required inservice education programs according to policies.

S – Attends all required inservice education programs according to policies.

A – Performs all behaviors described in S. Attends 90% of all inservice education programs offered for RNs.

E – Performs all behaviors described in A. When requested, actively participates in the planning and implementation of inservice programs. Recommends needed inservice programs. Actively participates with questions/comments/suggestions during the programs.

9. Formulates nursing prescriptions that delineate actions to be taken. Prescribed actions:

9.1 Are specific to the patient's problem and the desired outcomes;

9.2 Are based on scientific knowledge;

9.3 Are based on principles of patient teaching;

9.4 Are based on principles of psychosocial interactions;

9.5 Are based on environmental factors influencing the patient's health;

9.6 Include human, material, and community resources;

9.7 Include keeping patient knowledgeable of health status and total health care plan.

Explanation

After identifying patient problems and desired outcomes, the Registered Nurse prescribes actions to be taken in order to achieve desired outcomes. These actions are documented on the nursing care plan. The prescriptions include the seven criteria outlined above.

Evaluation Guide

U – Fails to meet the criteria outlined (9.1–9.7).

S – Satisfies all criteria outlined above and documents this within a 24-hour period.

A – Performs all behaviors described in S. Formulates and documents nursing prescriptions that delineate actions to be taken on all new admissions during that 8-hour shift.

E – Performs all behaviors described in A. From continual assessment and planning, adds to nursing prescriptions written from previous shifts on all assigned patients, each day.

10. Implements the actions delineated in the nursing prescription.

Actions Implemented

10.1 Actively involve the patient and family.

10.2 Are based on current scientific knowledge.

10.3 Are flexible and individualized for each patient.

10.4 Include principles of safety.

10.5 Include principles of infection control.

Explanation

> After formulating nursing prescription, the Registered Nurse implements the nursing actions delineated. All actions implemented are documented in the nurses' notes and reflect the total nursing care plan.

Evaluation Guide

U – Fails to meet the criteria outlined (10.1–10.5).

S – Satisfies all criteria outlined above and documents actions taken each shift.

A – Performs all behaviors described in S. Collaborates with physician and other members of the health care team in implementing actions.

E – Performs all behaviors described in A. Utilizes creative and innovative techniques in implementing actions. Involves staff in actions and teaches the rationale and scientific basis for the actions.

11. Conforms to hospital dress code (according to policy).

U – Seldom conforms to dress-code policy.

S – Usually conforms (90% of the time).

A – Always conforms to dress-code policy.

E – Is always immaculately dressed and groomed. Appears spotlessly clean, fresh, with shined shoes (and caps for females, as appropriate) at all times.

12. Is rarely sick or absent from work due to health.

Explanation

> Absenteeism is defined according to number of occurrences. An occurrence can be one day, or more days, related to a particular illness. For example, one "call-in" with the flu with two days of illness would be one occurrence. The supervisor counsels employees approaching six occurrences.

Evaluation Guide

U – Six occurrences.

S – Five occurrences. Always calls in advance according to policy.

A – Two to four occurrences per year.

E – One or no occurrences per year.

13. Is prompt and attends report (15 minutes prior to shift).

Evaluation Guide

U – Tardy six times per year.

S – Tardy five times. Always calls when knows will be late.

A – Tardy three to four times per year.

E – Tardy only two times per year or less.

Evaluation

1. Evaluates self-objectives, revises and formulates new objectives.

Explanation

The Registered Nurse evaluates her self-objectives to determine if the objectives have been achieved. She reassesses objectives to determine if they are realistic. From her evaluation, new or revised self-objectives are developed.

Evaluation Guide

U – Does not evaluate and revise self-objectives. Allows same objectives to continue month after month, with no improvement or change.

S – Evaluates achievement of self-objectives documented on evaluation form at the annual evaluation. Makes revisions and sets new objectives at this time.

A – Obtains input from peers and supervisory personnel when evaluating self-objectives. Provides rationale and pertinent facts to substantiate the evaluation of objectives. Documents objectives on evaluation form.

E – Performs all behaviors described in A. Evaluates, revises, and sets self-objectives every 3 months and maintains documentation of this evaluation.

2. Evaluates the effectiveness of problem-solving techniques and the activities implemented to improve nursing service.

Explanation

After the Registered Nurse has participated in planning methods to solve problems and implemented the plan, she evaluates the outcomes to determine if the problems have been solved. If the problem has not been solved, she reassesses the problem and actions taken and participates in determining new techniques to solve the problem. Other problems may also be identified by this evaluation.

Evaluation Guide

U – Never or rarely evaluates effectiveness of change or of problem-solving activities. Never notices improvement or effects of activities to improve nursing service.

S – When requested, will provide an evaluation of activities and problem-solving techniques. Can base evaluation on sound rationale with evidence of improvement.

A – Is self-motivated to evaluate nursing service activities. Communicates evidence substantiating evaluation of nursing service activities to supervisory personnel. Provides appropriate amount of time for planned change to occur before evaluating effectiveness of the change.

E – Performs all behaviors described in A. From evaluation, identifies new problems and new areas in need of work. Revises plan of action in accordance with the evaluation. Communicates this to supervisory personnel.

3. Contributes to the performance evaluations of nursing service personnel on the unit.

Explanation

The Registered Nurse provides input to the supervisor and head nurse concerning the performance of LPNs, NAs, and Unit Secretaries she works with directly on the unit.

Evaluation Guide

U – When asked, does not provide pertinent or substantial input to the supervisor concerning the performance of employees.

S – When asked, provides pertinent and substantial input concerning the employee's performance.

A – Performs all behaviors described in S. When asked, gives specific information concerning an employee's performance that indicates she is well aware of the quality of the performance, i.e., can give specific examples to substantiate her information.

E – Offers information to the supervisor for future evaluation of performance of employees she works with consistently, i.e., identifies above average performances as well as problem areas and need for improvement.

4. Participates in the evaluation of inservice education programs.

Explanation

The Registered Nurse provides input to the Inservice Director and supervisory personnel concerning appropriateness, content, and delivery of inservice education programs. The Registered Nurse communicates learning needs and whether these needs were met to the Inservice Director, following the program. The Registered Nurse identifies inservice needs and provides feedback concerning the utilization of the inservice on the unit. The Registered Nurse communicates ideas for improving the inservice programs.

Evaluation Guide

U – Never or rarely provides feedback concerning the need for inservice programs, or the utilization of information obtained from the inservice programs. Rarely evaluates the inservice education programs.

S – When asked, will communicate an evaluation of the inservice programs attended.

A – Is self-motivated to evaluate inservice programs and to communicate this evaluation. Bases evaluation on sound rationale. Identifies strengths and weaknesses of inservice programs and ways to utilize the knowledge gained on the unit.

E – Performs all behaviors described in A. Actively utilizes knowledge gained from inservices on the unit and evaluates the effectiveness of the actions. Recommends revisions in the program content from this evaluation. Requests clarification and explanations from the Inservice Director or supervisory personnel concerning content in programs and communicates ways to improve inservice offerings.

5. Evaluates achievement or lack of achievement of desired outcomes.

   5.1 Data are collected concerning the patient's health status.

   5.2 Data are compared to the specific desired outcomes.

5.3 The patient and nurse evaluate the achievement of desired outcomes.

Evaluation Guide

U – Fails to meet criteria (5.1–5.3).

S – Satisfies criteria listed above and documents achievement or lack of achievement of desired outcomes in nurses' notes.

A – Performs all behaviors described in S. Collaborates with the patient, health care team, and other personnel in evaluating achievement of desired outcomes. Discusses achievement or lack of achievement at shift report.

E – Performs all behaviors described in A. Includes assessment of slight alterations in the patient's health status and in the evaluation of achievement of desired outcomes.

6. From evaluation of achievement or lack of achievement of desired outcomes, reassesses and revises the nursing care plan:

   6.1 Reassesses the patient problems;

   6.2 Reassesses desired outcomes to determine if appropriate, realistic, and in correct priority;

   6.3 Reassesses nursing prescriptions to determine if appropriate, realistic, and stated accurately;

   6.4 Reassesses nursing actions for effectiveness in achieving desired outcomes.

   From reassessment:

   6.5 Determines new patient present/potential problems;

   6.6 From new patient problems, formulates and revises desired outcomes;

   6.7 Revises nursing prescriptions;

   6.8 Implements new actions in order to carry out revised prescriptions.

   6.9 Continually evaluates desired outcomes for achievement or lack of achievement;

   6.10 Continually evaluates and revises the nursing care plan according to changes in the patient's health status.

Evaluation Guide

U – Fails to meet criteria (6.1 to 6.10) and to document revisions in the nursing care plan.

S – Satisfies criteria listed above and documents revisions in the plan of care.

A – Gathers data from all possible sources and collaborates with all members of the health care team (as appropriate) in reassessing and revising the nursing care plan.

E – Reassesses and revises (as appropriate) the nursing care plan on all assigned patients each day and documents this on the nurses' notes and care plan each day.

APPENDIX 4-1
Annual Performance Evaluation Procedure

All new nursing service employees will be evaluated following their 3-month probationary period. The employee must score *satisfactory* on the evaluation in order to be removed from probation. If the employee does not meet job requirements, her probationary period will be extended for 1 additional month. If she meets job requirements (scores satisfactory), she will then be taken off probation and from this point evaluations will be performed annually. If the employee again does not meet job requirements (score satisfactory), she will be dismissed.

All nursing service employees will be evaluated annually according to the following ratings:

"U"—*Unsatisfactory*	"S"—*Satisfactory*	"A"—*Above average*	"E"—*Exceptional*
(Does not meet job requirements)	(Meets job requirements)	(Exceeds job requirements)	(Outstanding performance)

An employee scoring less than satisfactory will be placed on 3-months' probation. After 3 months, she will be reevaluated. If at this time the score is still unsatisfactory, she will be dismissed. If satisfactory, she is evaluated annually from this point.

An employee receiving a satisfactory score will receive across-the-board pay increase. Above average and exceptional employees receive raises according to the merit raise policy.

If the across-the-board pay increase occurs prior to or following an employee evaluation, it will then be given according to the last evaluation the employee received. All employees are eligible for the across-the-board pay increase unless they are on probation.

Evaluations will be performed according to the organizational chart. The Director of Nursing will evaluate the Supervisors and must review and sign all nursing service evaluations.

The Supervisors and Head Nurses will evaluate the nursing staff working on their respective shifts, units, and departments.

All items evaluated as "U" or "E" must have specific examples and reasons to justify the score.

Job descriptions that correlate with each evaluation with detailed criteria will be presented and kept available to all nursing service employees. Criteria used for evaluating performance according to categories U, S, A, and E will also be available to employees.

All employees will be continually monitored and advised by the Director of Nursing, Supervisors, and Head Nurses as to problem areas and need for improvement throughout the year. Evidence of employee's progress or lack of progress throughout the year will be documented by the Director of Nursing, Supervisors, and Head Nurses.

All employees will have a 6-month formal interviewing session by their immediate supervisor. This progress report will be signed and placed in the employee's file to be used at the annual evaluation time.

Employees will be provided with formal interview time during the year in order to receive feedback, ask questions, determine standing, and set goals for improvements.

Additional suggestions for improvement, recommended by the Supervisor or Head Nurse, should be documented on the last page of the evaluation.

The employee must document self-objectives at the 6-months and annual interview period.

Special needs, strengths, and weaknesses are written in the spaces provided under each item.

Any employee placed on extended probation will be counseled by the Director of Nursing. The Director of Nursing will also hold a dismissal interview on any employee that is dismissed.

An employee who is placed on probation for some reason related to attendance, tardiness, etc. will not receive the across-the-board raise or be eligible for a merit raise until taken off probation. An employee may also be placed on probation for the following reasons:

Evaluated as unsatisfactory (U) in any one area on a 6-month interview and again as unsatisfactory in that same area at the annual evaluation.

or

Evaluated as "U" in a specific area on the annual evaluation and again during the following 6-month interview.

then

After a 3-month probation, if the unsatisfactory area has not improved to "Satisfactory," the employee is dismissed. During this probation, the employee is given special inservice and counseling.

APPENDIX 4-2
Scoring Procedure

Following thorough investigation of existing methods of scoring, the committee developed this procedure. According to the committee, in order for an evaluation to be satisfactory at least 90% of the items on the performance evaluation must be rated as satisfactory. If not, the overall score would not adequately reflect the satisfactory achievement of the nursing standards. It was decided that for an above average score, at least 80% of all items should be rated as above average. The same was determined for excellent rating. Refer to the scoring procedure form at the end of each performance evaluation.

1. Add up all "U," "S," "A," and "E" scores. Write them in the blanks on the scoring sheet at the end of the evaluation form.
2. Multiply each total by the appropriate number. A "U" gets zero points, an "S" gets one point, an "A" receives two points, and an "E" receives three points.
3. The numbers are then tabulated and their sum equals the total score.
4. Compare this total score to the numbers comprising each rank. Wherever this number falls is the rank of that particular employee. For example, if "A" is 100–180, and the employee totaled a 160, she receives an above average rating.

The following is an example of how to develop the four ranking categories:

A particular performance evaluation has a total of 49 items. Multiply "49" in this way:

		U	S	A	E
$0 \times 49 =$	0 (U)	0 to 43	44 to 77	78 to 117	118 to 147
$1 \times 49 =$	49 (S)				
$2 \times 49 =$	98 (A)				
$3 \times 49 =$	147 (E)				

Then take the "S" number (49). Multiply it times 90% to receive 44.1. Because 0.1 is less than 5, it can be dropped. Write this number in the spot as indicated above. This is the minimum score that can be made to receive an S rating. Then take the "A" score, 98, and multiply it times 80% to receive 78.4. Again, the 0.4 is less than 5 and can be dropped. Write this number in the "A" spot as shown above. This becomes the minimum score that can be made to receive an above average rating. Anything less (77) becomes the top rank for the satisfactory level. Take the "E" total, 147, multiply it times 80% to receive 117.6. Because 0.6 is greater than 5, it raises the number to 118. This becomes the minimum score that can be made to receive an excellent rating. It is written in the first blank under E as shown above. Any number less falls into the A category as shown above. The top E score would indicate all items had received an excellent rating, or 3 points. This is derived by multiplying 3 times 49 items to equal 147. The U ranks from 0 to one point below satisfactory (43).

Each performance evaluation must be tabulated in the above manner, as each one (RN, LPN, Aide, etc.) has a different total of items. The scores are typed on the back of each form, made available at the nurse's stations, and used when evaluating their performance.

REFERENCES

1. Rosen, H., and Marella, M.: Basic quantitative thinking. JONA, May/June 1977, pp. 6–10.
2. Nyberg, J., and Simlee, M.: Developing a framework for an integrated nursing department. JONA, November 1979, pp. 9–15.
3. Alexander, E. L.: Nursing administration in the hospital health care system. St. Louis: C. V. Mosby Company, 1978, pp. 266–280.
4. Brief, A. P.: Developing a usable performance appraisal system. JONA, October 1979, pp. 7–10.
5. O'Loughlin, E. L., and Kaulbach, D.: Peer review: A perspective for performance appraisal. JONA, September 1981, pp. 22–27.
6. Christopher, W. I.: Management improvement for hospitals. St. Louis: W. I. Christopher & Associates, Inc., 1982.
7. Stevens, B. J.: The nurse as executive (2nd ed.). Wakefield, Mass.: Nursing Resources, Inc., 1980, pp. 303–325.
8. Engle, J. and Barkanskas, V.: The evolution of a public health nursing performance evaluation tool. JONA, April 1979, pp. 8–16.

BIBLIOGRAPHY

Boyar, D., Avery, J.: Peer review: Change and growth. Nurs. Admin. Quarterly, Winter 1981, (5), pp. 59–66.

Council, J. D., and Plachy, R. J.: Performance appraisal is not enough. JONA, October, 1980, pp. 20–25.

Cunningham, C. V.: Performance appraisal tests for staff nurses. Nurs. Times, May 1981, 28(77), pp. 61–3.

Curston, L. L.: Take the fat out of job evaluation. Health Serv. Manager, April 1981, (14), pp. 7–10.

Dyer, E. D., Cope, M., Monson, M.: Increasing the quality of patient care through performance counseling and written goal setting. Nurs. Res., 1975, 24(2), pp. 138–144.

Ganong, J., and Ganong, W.: Evaluating staff performance in current perspectives in nursing management (Vol. 1). Edited by Mariner, St. Louis: Mosby, 1979, pp. 56–69.

Golightly, C.: MBO and performance appraisal. JONA, September 1979, pp. 11–20.

Goodykoontz, L.: Performance evaluation of staff nurses. Supervisor Nurse, August 1981, (12), pp. 39–40.

Haar, L., and Hicks, J.: Performance appraisal. JONA, Spring 1976, pp. 20–29.

Jones, M. K., Lufkin, S. R.: Who wants to think about an unsatisfactory evaluation. Nursing, February 1981, (11), pp. 121–2.

Koerner, B. L.: Selected correlates of job performance of community health nurses. Nurs. Res., Jan/Feb 1981, (30), pp. 43–8.

McCaffrey, C.: Performance checklists: An effective method of teaching, learning and evaluating. Nurse Educator, January/February 1978, pp. 11–13.

Milner, R. F.: Performance analysis—Or how to. Supervisor Nurse, February 1981, (12), pp. 14–5.

Schlessberg, A.: Self-appraisal—A participative performance appraisal system. Nursing Homes, January/February 1981, (30), pp. 2–9.

5

Merit Raise System

Many organizational benefits are evident from the system described in the preceding chapters. Standards are maintained and mechanisms are instituted to correct deficiencies in employee behavior. But what about employee reward in this system? The employees understand the disadvantages of scoring unsatisfactory on the performance evaluation. What incentive do they have to improve above the satisfactory level? It would obviously improve the process of patient care and benefit the organization if all employees were either above average or excellent. What can be done to help motivate the employee to want to excel?

It is true that the employee must be self-motivated to improve, but certain reward procedures can be instituted that facilitate this self-motivation.[1] One such procedure is the system for providing merit raises.

PROS AND CONS

Merit raises as a motivator for improving performance are an interesting concept. Some authorities discuss monetary reward only as a satisfier of basic security needs. If the monetary reward is lacking, then the lower security needs are not satisfied.[2] When this happens, the morale can drop, leading to job dissatisfaction, and the employee cannot perform her work effectively. Monetary reward is not viewed as a primary motivation factor.[3] This viewpoint also maintains that higher needs, such as esteem and self-actualization, do not relate to money.

Herzberg states that money is a "hygienic factor" and in itself cannot motivate but can prevent serious decline in morale and productivity. This factor must be satisfied in order for other motivational factors to be effective. These other motivational factors are listed as recognition, achievement, advancement, and factors involving the type of work itself, including job responsibility.[3]

Other authorities believe that monetary rewards have some direct motivational effect on the employee. Knox[4] states that a system providing monetary rewards offers extrinsic motivation to the employee. Alexander[5] discusses many benefits from a fair and objective merit raise system. Employees feel more satisfaction towards their work and develop a sense of trust and equity toward the organization when compensated for good performance.

Watson's research revealed that the two factors influencing nurse retention in a job were administrative support and salary.[6] Kistler and Kistler state that there is a direct relationship between morale and wages. The employee evaluates her achievement of success according to her salary. Monetary rewards definitely help ensure improved employee performance.[1]

OTHER REWARD SYSTEMS

It is the general consensus that money alone does not motivate. Other reward systems must be present in addition to monetary reward.[7] For instance, some institutions are adapting clinical advancement programs. These programs clearly define job expectations for different levels of nursing practice. When the nurse is evaluated as achieving these expectations, she "graduates" to a higher clinical level and is recognized by the organization. She may receive a new title, such as RN II or RN III, and receive a raise and recognition from peers and her supervisor. This system stimulates motivation to improve without having to be promoted to a management position. It provides for advancement based on clinical performance and provides a reward system when certain expectations are achieved.[4]

Other types of reward systems involve the immediate supervisor's praise and recognition of the employee. This is important and often is overlooked by management personnel. To feel appreciated and needed is important in maintaining good morale and motivating the employee to continue to improve. Positive feedback can have a great effect on people. The organization as a whole can reward the employee, also. Some places have an employee-of-the-month award, or other types of recognition for employees. There are many types and ways to reward employees other than money.[8]

MONETARY REWARD SYSTEM

But money can facilitate the employee's motivation when used in combination with other types of rewards, such as those mentioned above. In order to motivate, the monetary reward system must include certain principles. The first principle is that a merit raise system is not tied into the yearly raises or across-the-board raises for all employees. If everyone receives the raise and it is not based on merit, the system will be meaningless and ineffective.[5] The system must also be understood and accepted by the employees. If it is not seen as fair, it will not work. There must be an objective, consistent mechanism for identifying and rewarding good performance; otherwise, it will produce negative repercussions and will destroy motivation.[9]

The key to the whole system is that it be linked to an effective and well accepted performance evaluation.[9] Only after effectively implementing and evaluating a system like the one described in the previous chapter should a merit raise system be initiated.

IMPLEMENTATION OF THE SYSTEM

The next step is how to get started. Obviously, there is no perfect way to begin. If the system is based on annual evaluations, all employees cannot be evaluated at one time. If they are evaluated each month, then in which month do you begin? This particular system was initiated in this way.

Nursing Service
Policy No. _____

Title: Merit Raise System

Approved
   by: Director of Nursing Service

Definition: A merit raise is a raise in salary awarded to an employee for performance exceeding job expectations. Because "satisfactory" rating is considered meeting job requirements, an "above-average" or "exceptional" rating is considered exceeding job expectations.

Procedure: All employees are eligible for a merit raise at the time of their annual performance evaluation. The total scoring on the performance evaluation will determine if a raise is awarded:

Unsatisfactory	Satisfactory	Above average	Exceptional
Does not meet job requirements	Meets job requirements	Exceeds job requirements	Outstanding performance
Probation	Across-the-board raises only	3% raise	5% raise

Merit raises are awarded as indicated above. Refer to the performance evaluation procedure for further information relating to the evaluation procedure.

Standard Policy   Issued: October 1982

Figure 5-1 A merit raise policy for nursing service.

A merit raise policy was written (see Figure 5-1). This defined the exact procedure to be implemented. Next, the hospital board voted to accept the policy and decided on the monetary increases to be awarded. Three percent was determined as the raise for above average, and 5% for excellent performance. All employees were inserviced on the policy. It was understood by all that only "above-average" and "excellent" performance would receive monetary reward. Satisfactory behavior means *meeting the job expectations* described in the job description. Only by *exceeding* job expectations is performance exceeding minimum requirements and, therefore, above the average.

All employees were then evaluated according to their anniversary dates. This was set up on a monthly basis and defined in the policy statement. The system was instituted in the month of October after a 6-month waiting period. This gave people time to discuss the policy and prepare for it. It also gave employees a chance to improve their performance in plenty of time before their evaluation.

The employees in July, August, and September were not very happy about the long wait but understood that it was done according to the date of employment. Because it was implemented in an objective way, with no exceptions, the employees accepted this. Management personnel were called upon to offer much support to employees during this time. The staff was allowed to vent feelings, discuss opinions, and offer ideas. But all in all, the employees were happy to be implementing this system.

The next problem to face was employees who were not happy with their scores. Before implementing the merit raise system, an "above average" or "excellent" rating did not have the same meaning to employees. Once money was tied into it, scoring higher became more important. For some reason, many employees felt they would automatically get a raise, or that simply by improving one month before their evaluation they would score above average. But this did not happen. One was quoted as saying, "You would think that just because I've been working here 20 years I would get a raise." It had to be constantly explained that only above-average performance merited a raise. Just by punching a time clock every day for 20 years does not mean that the work was being done well. An evaluation is based on the entire past year's performance. The management personnel needed much support in confronting these issues. It made them even more aware of the necessity of objectivity, feedback, and good documentation on the evaluations.

But a lot of good came out of the system. After about 6 months, employees who were improving and motivated were being rewarded monetarily for their efforts. Other employees who were "satisfactory" realized that they would not be compensated unless they improved. People started dressing and looking better, coming to work on time (and not missing as many days), and becoming much more interested in standards of nursing practice. Care plans improved and nurses were even asking questions about certain items on the job descriptions they had not been sure about. Even though the performance evaluation feedback had a mechanism for disciplining unsatisfactory behavior, a higher quality of performance had not been stimulated. After this system was implemented, a higher quality of work could be observed. Employees were asking ways they could improve. Even attendance at inservices was better. Nurses became very interested in achieving the criteria listed under the above-average and excellent ratings.

CONCLUSION

Again, money alone is not enough of a motivator to improve performance. But in combination with a good performance evaluation system and other mechanisms for reward, it could certainly help to improve performance. The merit raises can be said to have an indirect effect on this system. They help to stimulate improvement in employee performance. If this occurs, the standards of nursing practice are not simply minimally achieved but are carried out in a process that exceeds expectations. This can only lead to the provision of a higher quality of care.

REFERENCES

1. Kistler, J. F., and Kistler, R. C.: Motivation and morale in the hospital. Supervisor Nurse, Feb. 1980, (11), pp. 26–29.
2. Maslow, A.: Motivation and personality. New York: Harper and Row, 1954.
3. Herzberg, F.: Work and the nature of man. New York: World Publishing Co., 1966.
4. Knox, S.L.: A clinical advancement program. JONA, July 1980, (10), pp. 29–33.
5. Alexander, E.: Nursing administration in the hospital health care system (2nd ed.), St. Louis, C. V. Mosby Co., 1978, p. 274.
6. Watson, L.A.: Keeping qualified nurses, Supervisor Nurse, Oct. 1979, (10), pp. 29–31.
7. Jaski, E. B., Verre, M. O.: A systems approach to increased productivity. Supervisor Nurse, April 1981, (12), pp. 29–32.
8. Timmrock, T. C., and Randall, P. J.: Motivation, management and the supervisory nurse. Supervisor Nurse, March 1981, (12), pp. 28–31.
9. Stevens, B. J.: The nurse as executive (2nd ed.). Wakefield, Mass.: Nursing Resources, 1980.

BIBLIOGRAPHY

Evans, P. J.: Thinking of Maslow. Nursing Times, January 24, 1980, (76), pp. 163–165.
King, B. W.: Components of a motivation system: Communication. JEN, March/April 1981, (7), pp. 77–78.
King, B. W.: Motivation Theory. JEN, January/February 1981, (7), pp. 33–34.
Martin, G. G.: Staff motivation: Where do you start? MLO, March 1982, (14), p. 119.
National League for Nursing: Identifying problems in the motivation, performance and retention of nursing staff. Pub. No. 52-1802, NLN, 1979.

O'Connor, A. B., and Cantor, J.: Staff development: The problems of motivation. Journal of Continuing Ed. Nurs., March/April 1982, (13), pp. 10–14.

Ruskowski, U.: Recognize performance with merit increase (and keep your nurses happy), Dimens Health Serv., August 1981, (58), pp. 34–35.

Warren, J. C.: Motivating and rewarding the staff nurse. JONA, October 1978, (8), pp. 4–7.

6

The Nursing Quality Control System

A nursing department is an organization of activities that function as a quality control system. Its general purpose is to evaluate and monitor compliance with standards of nursing practice and to ensure optimal nursing care delivery. The system is composed of interrelated components or nursing activities that exist in a state of interdependence. For example, components or systems in nursing, such as staffing, depend on effective patient classification systems. Education and merit raise systems need effective nursing management systems to operate properly. Singly, these components have distinctive purposes and play individual roles in quality control activities. Together, they are utilized to maintain high standards for the hospital and ensure that optimal health care services are provided.[1] The management system described in this book is but one such component among several in the nursing quality control system.

Just as all activities in the nursing department exist for the same ultimate purpose, they must exchange data and channel these data into the data bank of the nursing quality assurance (NQA) committee. This is the core of the quality control system.[2] It is a centralized mechanism for receiving information from all systems, committees, and activities, directing the data appropriately and ensuring corrective action and continual improvement.[3] This nursing committee utilizes data from all the nursing and hospital-wide systems for the evaluation of nursing service.[4] It then feeds data back into the nursing activities or related hospital functions concerning evaluation results and need for corrective actions.[1] Figure 6-1 describes this process, and some of the nursing activities that feed into the system.

The nursing quality control system receives input, plans corrective actions, ensures the implementation of these actions, and evaluates and feeds results back into itself. the NQA committee receives input from all activities and functions in the nursing department. Data from nursing activities in functions such as pharmacy and therapeutics, medical records, and safety committee also feed

65

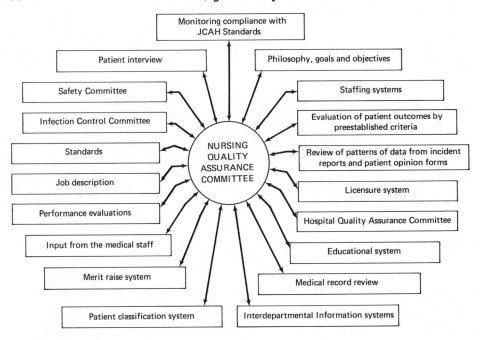

Figure 6-1 Nursing quality control system.

into this committee. It receives input from the hospital quality assurance committee, which is made up of all hospital departments. The NQA committee assesses information, identifies problems or potential problems concerning nursing services, and plans the appropriate action. It then channels this information as input into the appropriate nursing system for implementation. When the implementation is complete, the nursing system feeds the data back into the committee for evaluation. Evaluation data must be checked against the standards. The results are evaluated for effectiveness in problem solving, correcting deficiencies, and are monitored for resolution. Corrective actions may involve formal education, recommendations for changes in the operation of the hospital, or direct employee intervention.[5]

To illustrate further the concepts discussed, the following example is presented. Nursing education is a separate, self-contained system in the nursing department. It is also a component of the nursing quality control system. Some of its purposes are to identify educational needs among the staff, to provide classes and instruction, and to promote continual intellectual growth and development of skills. Nursing education contributes to quality assurance—improving employee performance by increasing expertise and knowledge levels, thus improving the quality of services.[6] Problems identified in the nursing quality assurance committee may enter into the educational system for corrective action by inservice education. Feedback from the educational system enters the reports to the quality assurance committee concerning needs identified from classes that affect other systems or results from educational offerings that reflect improvement in patient care.

The management system described in this book works in the same manner within the quality control system. When operating properly, it reflects compliance with nursing standards. It also reflects compliance with job descriptions, effectiveness of management skills in improving quality of nursing processes, and the effectiveness of other systems, such as education in teaching skills related to nursing standards and job performance. All of this evaluation information is fed into the data bank of the quality assurance committee, to be confirmed by data received from other systems. If the educational system indicates, for example, that nurses have improved on patient care planning in the classroom and demonstrate expertise in writing care plans, data from the performance evaluation results should be consistent. The items on the performance evaluation concerning patient care planning may have scores of above average or excellent, indicating expertise in this area. All activities, systems, and functions in the nursing department must be considered in the evaluation of quality care. One system alone is not sufficient.[2]

Data from various sources are utilized to indicate quality care. For instance, in the above example of patient care planning, other data are needed to validate results. For example, nursing is represented on safety committee and collects data about patient safety. Patterns can be determined from these data that reflect problem areas. These problems are fed into nursing quality assurance committee information pool for further assessment. A pattern may show, for instance, that patients falling out of bed had been suffering from disorientation. Further assessment determines that over a period of several days the patients had become confused, tried to climb out of bed, and had fallen. After thorough investigation, the problem is finally identified as incomplete patient care planning. Investigation reveals that the assessment phase of the nursing process was complete, but once the problem of disorientation was identified it was not integrated into the patients' plan of care. Evaluation results from education and management systems concerning patient care planning feed into the quality assurance committee information system along with data from the safety committee. An obvious discrepancy is identified among the systems. This discrepancy serves as input into the educational system for further inservicing of patient care planning. It also is input into the management system for correction of noncompliance with the nursing standards concerning both safety and patient care planning. Standards, job descriptions, and performance evaluations may be reviewed to ensure that this aspect of safety is clear and specific. Performance evaluation techniques may be monitored for correctness and for accurate data collection. Even safety policies may be revised. It is seen that when a problem exists it may show up in one system, but affect two or three other systems, and the corrective action may do the same. Most importantly, feedback from all systems must be centralized so that data are appropriately utilized.[7] Only when data from all related sources indicate a quality evaluation can quality of services be assured. That is why data from all systems and activities must be continually monitored.

Just as nursing process is the theoretical foundation for our nursing management system, it is also the basis for the nursing quality control system. Findings from the infection control committee illustrate this point.

Information involving increased occurrence of urinary tract infection is identified by the infection control committee. The problem is assessed and identified as noncompliance with infection control standards specifically related to the insertion and care of urinary catheters. The desired outcome is determined and the corrective action is planned.

In this case, planning again includes nursing management and education systems. In the management system, it concerns aspects such as orientation and appropriate supervision, input to employees during their performance evaluations, and correction of noncompliance with the nursing infection control standards. Reorienting these employees to procedures and teaching appropriate technique involves the educational system. Carrying out the planned corrective actions is the implementation phase in the nursing quality control system. Several systems may work together to implement the corrective actions.

Afterwards the results from the implementation phase are evaluated. Results from performance evaluations, observations, supervision, and inservice classes feed into reports to the nursing quality assurance committee. Then data from infection control committee may be recollected and reports monitored for results. If the reports and data indicate the problem is solved (according to the pre-established criteria), these data feed back into the management and education systems, confirming their results. It may be that the problem is reassessed at a later date to ensure that it has been solved. Again, data from several sources must be collected in order to evaluate accurately the quality of services being delivered.[8]

On the other hand, data from infection control committee may have reflected very low infection rates throughout the patient population. Along with other data, infection control standards can be accurately evaluated for compliance. Surveillance activities by supervisors may indicate good sterile technique by nurses when inserting catheters. The performance evaluation results concerning infection control activities may be above average or excellent ratings. These data collectively can be utilized as valid indicators of compliance with nursing standards in the areas relating to infection control practices.

In implementing the system presented in this book, the reader must keep in mind that this is but one component in the nursing quality control system. Its purpose, as stated earlier, is to indicate nursing service's compliance with standards of nursing practice. In coordination with the other activities in the nursing department, however, this system can contribute to the evaluation process and be a valid indicator of quality patient care.

REFERENCES

1. Stevens, B. J.: The nurse as executive. Wakefield, Mass.: Nursing Resources (2nd ed.). 1980, pp. 287–301.

2. Tan, M. W.: Quality Assurance in Nursing, Seminar Manual. Chicago, Illinois; Inter-Qual 1980, pp. 55–57.

3. Marriner, A.: The research process in quality assurance. AJN Dec. 1979, 79(12), pp. 2158–2161.

4. Lindy, C. N.: A three-part approach to quality assurance in nursing. QRB, March 1980, 6(3), pp. 12–16.

5. Slee, V. N.: How to know if you have quality control. Hospital Progress. 1972, 53(1), pp. 38–43.

6. Kaplan, K. O. and Hopkins, J. M.: The QA Guide, a Resource for Hospital Quality Assurance. Chicago, Illinois: The Joint Commission, 1980, pp. 119–124.

7. Graham, N. O.: Quality Assurance in Hospitals: Strategies for Assessment and Implementation. Rockville, Maryland: Aspen Systems, 1982, pp. 285–287.

8. Sabatino, F. G.: Principles of quality assurance. QRB Special Edition, 1979, pp. 4–7.

BIBLIOGRAPHY

Barney, M.: Measuring quality of patient care: A computerized approach. Supervisor. Nurse, May 1981, (12), pp. 40–44.

Block, D.: Evaluation of nursing care in terms of process and outcome: Issues in research and quality assurance. Nur. Res., July/Aug. 1975, (24), pp. 256–263.

Bloomrosen, M.: The development of a quality control program: Activity reporting and performance standards; JAM Med. Rec. Assoc., Aug. 1980, (51), pp. 37–63.

Donabedian, A.: Promoting quality through evaluating the process of patient care, Medical Care, VI(3), May/June 1968, pp. 181–202.

Grahm, N. O.: Quality assurance in hospitals; Strategies for assessment and implementation, Rockville, Maryland: Aspen Systems, 1982.

Kuehnel, C., Rowe, B.: Patient education and the audit . . . a new format developed for a teaching Kardex. Supervisor Nurse, Dec. 1980, (11), pp. 15–19.

National League for Nursing. Criteria for departments of nursing in long-term care settings: A guide for self-appraisal (20-1830 Pub. No.) NLN Publ. Div. Hosp. Long-term Care Nurs. Serv. 1980, pp. 1–85.

National League for Nursing Quality Assessment: Program and process, Pub. No. 52-1598; NLN, 1975.

Phaneaf, M. C., Wandeit, M. A.: Three methods of process-oriented nursing evaluation, QRB, Aug. 1981, (7), pp. 20–26.

Rinaldi, L. A.: Quality assurance '81—Satisfying JCAH: What does compliance to the new standards mean? Nurs. Manage. Sept. 1981, (12), pp. 23–24.

Sebatino, F.: Toward a comprehensive quality assurance program. QRB Special Ed. 1979, pp. 2–3.

Shaffer, K. L., Linderstein, J., and Jennings, T. A.: Successful QA program incorporates new JCAH standard. Hospitals, Aug. 1981, 16(55), pp. 117–118.

7

Medical-Surgical Nursing Practice

STANDARDS OF MEDICAL-SURGICAL NURSING PRACTICE

STANDARD I

Assessment is the identification and gathering of data concerning the health status of the patient. This process is complete, continuous, and systematic as evidenced by:

1. *A comprehensive patient history and physical:*
   a. *Patient interview*
      Chief complaint
      History of present illness
      Allergies
      Medications
      Past medical history
      Cultural, environmental, and socioeconomic conditions
      Activities of daily living
      Personal habits
      Food and fluid preferences
      Appetite changes/weight changes
      Available and accessible human, community, and material resources
   b. *Psychological assessment*
      Emotional status
      Patterns of coping
      Concerns during hospitalization
   c. *Physical assessment*
      Personal hygiene and grooming
      Nutritional status
      Mental status
      Physical status
   d. *Perception of illness*
      Understanding of disease process/illness
      Understanding of reasons for hospitalization
      Desired outcome from hospitalization
2. *The collection of data from available sources:*
   Patient, family, significant other
   Health care providers
   Individuals and/or agencies in the community
3. *The collection of data by scientific methodology:*
   Interview
   Observation
   Inspection
   Ausculation
   Palpation
   Reports and records
4. *The organization of data in a systematic arrangement:*
   The arrangement provides:

Accurate collection
Complete collection
Accessibility
Confidentiality
5. *The communication of data in an orderly fashion:*
Data are recorded by each shift, daily.
Data are updated by each shift, daily.
Data are revised and recorded as appropriate.
Data are communicated verbally among health team, daily.

STANDARD II

Nursing care planning consists of determining patient problems and desired outcomes. Planning involves preparing the patient for home care. This is evidenced by:

1. *The identification of present/potential patient problems, from the patient assessment:*
Data are grouped into meaningful arrangement, based upon scientific knowledge.
Patient's health status is determined.
Patient's health status is compared to the norms.
Present and potential problems are identified.
Problems are given priority according to impact upon the patient's health status.
2. *The formulation of desired outcomes:*
Patient (family, significant other) and nurse mutually agree upon the patient's present/potential health problems.
Patient and nurse mutually agree upon desired outcomes.
Desired outcomes are congruent with the patient problems and established norms.
Desired outcomes are specific.
Desired outcomes are measureable within a certain time frame.
Desired outcomes are consistent with other health provider's expectations.
Desired outcomes are established to restore patient's optimal functioning capabilities.
3. *The incorporation of home health care into desired outcomes involves teaching:*
Disease process and complications
Medication
Diet
Exercise/activity
Self-care techniques and materials
Available support systems and resources

STANDARD III

The plan of care is implemented in order to achieve the desired outcome. This is evidenced by:

1. *The formulation of nursing prescriptions that delineate actions to be taken: Prescribed actions:*
   Are specific to identified patient problems and desired outcomes.
   Are based on current scientific knowledge.
   Incorporate principles of patient teaching.
   Incorporate principles of psychosocial interactions.
   Incorporate environmental factors influencing the patient's health.
   Include human, material, and community resources.
   Include keeping patient knowledgeable of health status and total health care plan.

2. *The implementation of actions delineated in the nursing prescriptions: Actions implemented:*
   Actively involve the patient and family.
   Are consistent with the nursing prescriptions.
   Are based upon current scientific knowledge.
   Are flexible and individualized for each patient.
   Include principles of safety.
   Include principles of infection control.

STANDARD IV

Outcomes of Nursing Actions are evaluated for further assessment and planning. This is evidenced by:

1. *Evaluating the achievement of desired outcomes:*
   Data are collected concerning the patient's health status.
   Data are compared to the specified desired outcomes.
   The patient and nurse evaluate the achievement of desired outcomes.

2. *Reassessment of the nursing care plan:*
   Outcome of nursing actions direct the reassessment of identified patient problems.
   Outcome of nursing actions direct assessment of desired outcomes (assess the desired outcome to determine if appropriate, realistic, and in correct priority).
   Outcome of nursing actions direct reassessment of nursing prescriptions (assess the nursing prescriptions to determine if appropriate, realistic, and stated accurately).
   Nursing actions are assessed for effectiveness in achieving desired outcomes.

3. *Further planning as directed by the reassessment:*
   Reassessment determines new patient present/potential problems.
   New patient problems direct the formulation and revision of desired outcomes.
   Revised desired outcomes direct new actions to be implemented toward desired outcomes.
   Desired outcomes are continually evaluated for achievement.
   The plan of care is continually evaluated and revised according to changes in the patient's health status.

MEDICAL-SURGICAL SUPERVISOR (DAY SHIFT): JOB DESCRIPTION

Position Requirements: Graduate from an accredited school of nursing with current licensure as a registered nurse in the State of Alabama. Five years recent clinical experience, including at least 1 year supervisory experience.

Professional Requirements: Pursues programs of continuing education consistent with requirements of Alabama Nurses' Association. Participates in educational conferences and updates and maintains professional knowledge and skills related to the management of areas of responsibility.

Position Accountable for: All nursing care behaviors described in the Medical-Surgical Supervisor Day Shift (Assistant Director) job description.

Position Accountable to: Director of Nursing Service, the patient, and family.

Position Summary: Performs the primary functions of a professional nurse leader in assessing, planning, directing, and evaluating patient care on a 24-hour basis. Is responsible for meeting the Joint Commission Standards of Nursing Practice; for managing all personnel, supplies and equipment on the units, and for promoting teamwork with physicians and personnel of other departments.

In the absence of the Director of Nursing Service, assumes responsibility for direction of patient care and makes immediate administrative decisions for the entire nursing service, utilizing knowledge of standards, policies, and procedures outlined for the hospital.

I. *Assessment*
   1. Assesses the number and level of personnel needed to provide quality patient care and adjusts staffing and assignments appropriately.
   2. Assesses the delivery of nursing care and identifies problems and any need for improvements.
   3. Assesses the health status of patients on a daily basis, as outlined in nursing standards. Ensures that:

3.1 A comprehensive history and physical including patient interview, psychological and physical assessment, as well as patient's perception of illness is completed on each patient.

3.2 Data are collected from the patient, family and significant others, health care providers, individuals, and/or agencies in the community.

3.3 Data are collected by: interview, observation, inspection, auscultation, palpation, and reports and records.

3.4 Assessment data are organized so that they are accurate, complete, accessible, and remain confidential.

3.5 Assessment data are communicated in an orderly fashion among the health team daily, recorded, updated, and revised appropriately.

II. *Planning*

1. Serves on hospital committees, revises and recommends policies and procedures that effect overall hospital operations.

2. Plans and develops self-objectives.

3. Plans ways to solve problems and to make improvements in the delivery of patient care in collaboration with the Director of Nursing.

4. Ensures that all patients have a nursing care plan. Establishes individual patient's care plans as well as directs and supervises others in the formulation of patient care plans. Ensures that:

   4.1 The patient's present/potential problems are identified from the patient assessment.

      a. patient's health status is determined,

      b. health status is compared to the norms,

      c. problems are given priority according to impact upon the patient's health status.

   4.2 Desired outcomes are formulated specific to the patient problems and established norms.

   4.3 Desired outcomes are mutually agreed upon by the patient and nurse and are: (a) specific, (b) measurable within a certain time frame, and (c) consistent with other health provider's expectations.

   4.4 Home health care is incorporated into the patient's desired outcomes. This includes but is not limited to teaching about the disease process and complications, medications, diet, exercise/activity, self-care techniques and materials, and available support systems and resources.

III. *Implementation*

1. Implements activities necessary to meeting self-objectives.

2. Promotes the achievement of nursing service objectives.

3. Directs, supervises, and participates in implementing planned changes and activities to improve nursing service in collaboration with the Director of Nursing.

4. Ensures that the Medical-Surgical Standards of Nursing Practice are implemented and assists in monitoring of standards as necessary.

5. Holds self and staff accountable for the delivery of quality nursing care.

6. Acts rapidly and effectively, follows hospital policies and procedures, and utilizes principles of management, in any emergency situation.

7. Promotes harmonious relationships and favorable attitudes among the health care team.

8. Interprets, supports, and recommends administrative and nursing service policies and procedures for employees. Applies knowledge and skills of management.

9. Directs and assists with orientation of new employees.

10. Keeps the Director of Nursing Service informed on reportable situations and nursing unit needs.

11. Attends required inservice education programs.

12. Ensures that nursing prescriptions are formulated as outlined in the Nursing Standard, which delineate actions to be taken. Ensures that prescribed actions:
    12.1 Are specific to the patient's problems and the desired outcomes.
    12.2 Are based on scientific knowledge.
    12.3 Incorporate principles of patient teaching.
    12.4 Incorporate principles of psychosocial interactions.
    12.5 Incorporate environmental factors influencing the patient's health.
    12.6 Include human, material, and community resources.
    12.7 Include keeping patient knowledgeable of health status and total health care plan.

13. Ensures that the actions delineated in the nursing prescriptions are implemented. Actions implemented:
    13.1 Actively involve the patient and family.
    13.2 Are based on current scientific knowledge.
    13.3 Are flexible and individualized for each patient.
    13.4 Include principles of safety.
    13.5 Include principles of infection control.

14. Serves as consultant in technical and professional matters for personnel.

15. Participates and contributes to a unified Quality Assurance Program.

16. Conforms to hospital dress code.

17. Is rarely sick or absent from work due to health.

18. Is prompt and attends report.

IV. *Evaluation*

1. Continually evaluates Medical-Surgical Standards of Nursing Practice by reviewing nursing care plans, assessing patients, reviewing charts, interviewing, observing, participating in Quality Assurance activities, and employing other means of evaluation. Participates in revision of standards as appropriate.

2. Evaluates policies and procedures and recommends the need for revision.

3. Evaluates self-objectives and determines need for revision and new objectives.

4. Evaluates the effectiveness of problem-solving techniques and activities implemented to improve nursing service.
5. Evaluates the performance of nursing service personnel.
6. Evaluates the achievement of nursing service objectives in collaboration with Director of Nursing.
7. Evaluates emergencies and any hospital disaster and recommends revisions in policies and procedures and/or need for improvement in employee performance.
8. Evaluates orientation policies and procedures and recommends revisions as necessary.
9. Evaluates inservice education programs.
10. Ensures that desired outcomes are evaluated for achievement or lack of achievement.
    10.1 Data are collected concerning the patient's health status.
    10.2 Data are compared to the specific desired outcomes.
    10.3 The patient and nurse evaluate the achievement of desired outcomes.
11. Ensures that the nursing care plans are reassessed and revised according to the evaluation of achievement or lack of achievement of desired outcomes.

    From evaluation:
    11.1 Reassesses the patient problems.
    11.2 Reassesses desired outcomes to determine if appropriate, realistic, and in correct priority.
    11.3 Reassesses nursing prescriptions to determine if appropriate, realistic, and stated accurately.
    11.4 Reassesses nursing actions for effectiveness in achieving desired outcomes.

    From reassessment:
    11.5 New patient present/potential problems are determined.
    11.6 From new patient problems, desired outcomes are formulated and revised.
    11.7 Nursing prescriptions are revised.
    11.8 New actions are implemented in order to carry out revised prescriptions.
    11.9 Desired outcomes are continually evaluated for achievement or lack of achievement.
    11.10 The nursing care plan is continually evaluated and revised according to changes in the patient's health status.

MEDICAL-SURGICAL SUPERVISOR (DAY SHIFT): PERFORMANCE EVALUATION

Name _____ Employment Date _____

Rating Period _____ To _____

Department _____ Job Title _____

Instructions: Using the following rating scale, indicate the quality of performance by placing the appropriate letter on the line to the left of the item.

U* – Unsatisfactory (does not meet job requirements)
S – Satisfactory (meets job requirements)
A – Above average (exceeds job requirements)
E* – Exceptional performance

I. *Assessment:*

_____ 1. Assesses the number and level of personnel needed to provide quality patient care and adjusts staffing and assignments appropriately.

_____

_____

_____ 2. Assesses the delivery of nursing care and identifies problems and any need for improvements.

_____

_____

_____ 3. Assesses the health status of patients on a daily basis, as outlined in the nursing standards. Ensures that:
   3.1 A comprehensive history and physical including patient interview, psychological and physical assessment, as well as patient's perception of illness is completed on each patient.

_____

_____

   3.2 Data are collected from the patient, family and significant others, health care providers, individuals, and/or agencies in the community.

_____

_____

---

*The evaluator is expected to comment on all items rated "U" or "E."

3.3 Data are collected by: interview, observation, inspection, auscultation, palpation, and reports and records.

_____

_____

3.4 Assessment data are organized so that they are accurate, complete, and accessible, and so that they remain confidential.

_____

_____

3.5 Assessment data are communicated in an orderly fashion among the health team daily and are recorded, updated, and revised appropriately.

_____

_____

II. *Planning:*

_____ 1. Serves on hospital committees, revises and recommends policies and procedures that affect overall hospital operations.

_____

_____

_____ 2. Plans and develops self-objectives.

_____

_____

_____ 3. Plans ways to solves problems and to make improvements in the delivery of patient care in collaboration with the Director of Nursing.

_____

_____

_____ 4. Ensures that all patients have a nursing care plan. Establishes individual patient's care plans as well as directs and supervises others in the formulation of patient care plans. Ensures that:
   4.1 The patient's present/potential problems are identified from the patient assessment.
       a. patient's health status is determined,
       b. health status is compared to the norms,
       c. problems are given priority according to impact upon the patient's health status.

_____

_____

4.2 Desired outcomes are formulated specific to the patient problems and established norms.

_____

_____

4.3 Desired outcomes are mutually agreed upon by the patient and nurse and are: (a) specific, (b) measurable within a certain time frame, and (c) consistent with other health provider's expectations.

_____

_____

4.4 Home health care is incorporated into the patient's desired outcomes. This includes but is not limited to teaching about the disease process and complications, medications, diet, exercise/activity, self-care techniques and materials, and available support systems and resources.

_____

_____

III. _Implementation:_

_____ 1. Implements activities necessary to meeting self-objectives.

_____

_____

_____ 2. Promotes the achievement of nursing service objectives.

_____

_____

_____ 3. Directs, supervises, and participates in implementing planned changes and activities to improve nursing service in collaboration with the Director of Nursing.

_____

_____

_____ 4. Ensures that the Medical-Surgical Standards of Nursing Practice are implemented and assists in monitoring of standards as necessary.

_____

_____

_____ 5. Holds self and staff accountable for the delivery of quality nursing care.

_____

_____

_____ 6. Acts rapidly and effectively, follows hospital policies and procedures, and utilizes principles of management in any emergency situation.

_____

_____

_____ 7. Promotes harmonious relationships and favorable attitudes among the health care team.

_____

_____

_____ 8. Interprets, supports, and recommends administrative and nursing service policies and procedures for employees. Applies knowledge and skills of management.

_____

_____

_____ 9. Directs and assists with orientation of new employees.

_____

_____

_____ 10. Keeps the Director of Nursing Service informed on reportable situations and nursing unit needs.

_____

_____

_____ 11. Attends required inservice education programs.

_____

_____

_____ 12. Ensures that nursing prescriptions are formulated as outlined in the Nursing Standard, which delineate actions to be taken. Ensures that the prescribed actions:

12.1 Are specific to the patient's problems and the desired outcomes.

_____

_____

12.2 Are based on scientific knowledge.

_____

_____

12.3 Incorporate principles of patient teaching.

_____

_____

12.4 Incorporate principles of psychosocial interactions.

_____

_____

12.5 Incorporate environmental factors influencing the patient's health.

_____

_____

12.6 Include human, material, and community resources.

_____

_____

12.7 Include keeping patient knowledgeable of health status and total health care plan.

_____

_____

_____ 13. Ensures that actions delineated in the nursing prescriptions are implemented. Actions implemented:

13.1 Actively involve the patient and family.

_____

_____

13.2 Are based on current scientific knowledge.

_____

_____

13.3 Are flexible and individualized for each patient.

_____

_____

13.4 Include principles of safety.

_____

_____

13.5 Include principles of infection control.

_____

_____

_____ 14. Serves as consultant in technical and professional matters for personnel.

_____

_____

_____ 15. Participates and contributes to a unified Quality Assurance Program.

_____

_____

_____ 16. Conforms to hospital dress code.

_____

_____

_____ 17. Is rarely sick or absent from work due to health.

_____

_____

_____ 18. Is prompt and attends report.

_____

_____

IV. *Evaluation:*

_____ 1. Continually evaluates Medical-Surgical Standards of Nursing Practice by reviewing nursing care plans, assessing patients, reviewing charts, interviewing, observing, participating in Quality Assurance activities, and employing other means of evaluation. Participates in revision of standards as appropriate.

_____

_____

_____ 2. Evaluates policies and procedures and recommends the need for revision.

_____

_____

_____ 3. Evaluates self-objectives and determines need for revision and new objectives.

_____

_____

_____ 4. Evaluates the effectiveness of problem-solving techniques and activities implemented to improve nursing service.

_____

_____

_____ 5. Evaluates the performance of nursing service personnel.

_____

_____

_____ 6. Evaluates the achievement of nursing service objectives in collaboration with Director of Nursing.

_____

_____

_____ 7. Evaluates emergencies and any hospital disaster and recommends revisions in policies and procedures and/or need for improvement in employee performance.

_____

_____

_____ 8. Evaluates orientation policies and procedures and recommends revisions as necessary.

_____

_____

_____ 9. Evaluates inservice education programs.

_____

_____

_____ 10. Ensures that desired outcomes are evaluated for achievement or lack of achievement.
10.1 Data are collected concerning the patient's health status.

_____

10.2 Data are compared to the specific desired outcomes.

_____

10.3 The patient and nurse evaluate the achievement of desired outcomes.

_____

_____

_____ 11. Ensures that the nursing care plans are reassessed and revised according to the evaluation of achievement or lack of achievement of desired outcomes.

From evaluation:
11.1 Reassesses the patient problems.

_____

11.2 Reassesses desired outcomes to determine if appropriate, realistic, and in correct priority.

_____

_____

11.3 Reassesses nursing prescriptions to determine if appropriate, realistic, and stated accurately.

_____

_____

11.4 Reassesses nursing actions for effectiveness in achieving desired outcomes.

_____

_____

From reassessment:

11.5 New patient present/potential problems are determined.

_____

_____

11.6 From new patient problems desired outcomes are formulated and revised.

_____

_____

11.7 Nursing prescriptions are revised.

_____

_____

11.8 New actions are implemented in order to carry out revised prescriptions.

_____

_____

11.9 Desired outcomes are continually evaluated for achievement or lack of achievement.

_____

_____

11.10 The nursing care plan is continually evaluated and revised according to changes in the patient's health status.

_____

_____

MEDICAL-SURGICAL SUPERVISOR: SCORING PROCEDURE

Instructions: Total the number of each item and multiply times the appropriate number. Add these totals to make the score.

U _____ × 0 = _____

S _____ × 1 = _____

A _____ × 2 = _____

E _____ × 3 = _____   _____ Total Score

Compare total score to the following scale to determine rank:

U	S	A	E
0 to 31	32 to 57	58 to 85	86 to 108

Overall Performance Review Score _____.

ALL ITEMS IN THE FOLLOWING SECTION MUST BE COMPLETED:

A. Interviewer's comments on overall review _____

_____

_____

B. Additional suggestions for overall work improvement and goals for next evaluation _____

_____

_____

_____

C. Self-objectives _____

_____

_____

_____

_____   _____

Date   Employee's signature

_____   _____

Date   Interviewer's signature

_____   _____

Date   Director of Nursing

MEDICAL-SURGICAL REGISTERED NURSE: JOB DESCRIPTION

Position Requirements:	Graduate from an accredited school of nursing with current licensure as a registered nurse in the state of Alabama.
Professional Requirements:	Pursues programs of continuing education consistent with requirements of the Alabama Nurses' Association, participates in educational conferences, and updates and maintains professional knowledge and skills related to areas of responsibilities.
Position Accountable for:	All nursing care behaviors described in the Medical-Surgical RN job description.
Position Accountable to:	Head Nurse, Supervisor, Director of Nursing, the patient, and family.
Position Summary:	Performs the primary functions of an RN in assessing, planning implementing, and evaluating the care of all assigned patients on the unit during her shift. Is responsible for meeting the established Medical-Surgical Standards of Nursing Practice, for managing all assigned personnel, supplies and equipment on the unit, and for promoting team work with physicians and personnel of other departments.

I. *Assessment*
   1. Assesses the number and level of personnel needed to provide quality patient care on the unit and collaborates with the Head Nurse or Supervisor in adjusting staffing and assignments.
   2. Assesses the delivery of nursing care on the unit and identifies problems and any need for improvements.
   3. Assesses the health status of assigned patients on the unit as outlined in the nursing standards.
      3.1 Completes a comprehensive patient history and physical including patient interview, psychological and physical assessment, as well as patient's perception of illness.
      3.2 Collects data from the patient, family and significant others, health care providers, individuals, and/or agencies in the community.
      3.3 Collects data by: interview, observation, inspection, auscultation, palpation, and reports and records.
      3.4 Organizes assessment data so that they are accurate, complete, accessible, and so that they remain confidential.
      3.5 Communicates assessment data in an orderly fashion by recording,

updating, and communicating among the health team daily and revising as appropriate.

II. *Planning*

1. Serves on hospital committees and helps to review and revise policies and procedures, as directed by Head Nurse or Supervisor.
2. Plans and develops self-objectives.
3. Plans ways to solve problems and to make improvements on the unit in collaboration with supervisory personnel.
4. Completes a written care plan for assigned patients on the unit. Plans the care for individual patients as well as directs and supervises others in the planning of patient's care.
   4.1 Identifies the patient's present/potential problems from the patient assessment.
       a. patient's health status is determined,
       b. health status is compared to the norms,
       c. problems are given priority according to impact upon the patient's health status.
   4.2 Formulates desired outcomes specific to the patient problems and established norms.
   4.3 Ensures that desired outcomes are mutually agreed upon by the patient and nurse and are: (a) specific, (b) measureable within a certain time frame, and (c) consistent with other health provider's expectations.
   4.4 Incorporates home health care into the patient's desired outcomes. This includes but is not limited to teaching about the disease process and complications, medications, diet, exercise/activity, self-care techniques and materials, and available support systems and resources.

III. *Implementation*

1. Implements activities necessary to meeting self-objectives.
2. Participates in implementing planned changes and activities to improve nursing service.
3. Holds self accountable for the delivery of quality nursing care.
4. Promotes harmonious relationships and favorable attitudes among the health care team.
5. Supports and adheres to administrative and nursing service policies and procedures.
6. Assists with orientation of new employees.
7. Acts rapidly and effectively, manages self, patients, and other employees during any emergency situation.
8. Attends required inservice education programs.
9. Formulates nursing prescriptions that delineate actions to be taken. Prescribed actions:
   9.1 Are specific to the patient's problems and the desired outcomes.
   9.2 Are based on scientific knowledge.

9.3 Are based of principles of patient teaching.

9.4 Are based on principles on psychosocial interactions.

9.5 Are based on environmental factors influencing the patient's health.

9.6 Include human, material, and community resources.

9.7 Include keeping patient knowledgeable of health status and total health care plan.

10. Implements the actions delineated in the nursing prescriptions. Actions implemented:

10.1 Actively involve the patient and family.

10.2 Are based on current scientific knowledge.

10.3 Are flexible and individualized for each patient.

10.4 Include principles of safety.

10.5 Include principles of infection control.

11. Conforms to hospital dress code.

12. Is rarely sick or absent from work due to health.

13. Is prompt and attends report.

IV. *Evaluation*

1. Evaluates self-objectives, revises and formulates new objectives.

2. Evaluates the effectiveness of problem-solving techniques and the activities implemented to improve nursing service.

3. Contributes to the performance evaluation of nursing service personnel on the unit.

4. Participates in evaluation of RN orientation policies and procedures and recommends revisions to Supervisor or Head Nurse.

5. Participates in the evaluation of inservice education programs.

6. Evaluates achievement or lack of achievement of desired outcomes.

6.1 Data are collected concerning the patient's health status.

6.2 Data are compared to the specific desired outcomes.

6.3 Includes the patient's evaluation of the achievement of desired outcomes.

6.4 Reassesses nursing actions for effectiveness in achieving desired outcomes.

7. From evaluation of achievement or lack of achievement of desired outcomes, reassesses and revises the nursing care plan.

From evaluation:

7.1 Reassesses the patient problems.

7.2 Reassesses desired outcomes to determine if appropriate, realistic, and in correct priority.

7.3 Reassesses nursing prescriptions to determine if appropriate, realistic, and stated accurately.

From reassessment:

7.4 Determines new patient present/potential problems.

7.5 From new patient problems, formulates and revises desired outcomes.

7.6 Revises nursing prescriptions.

7.7 Implements new actions in order to carry out revised prescriptions.

7.8 Continually evaluates desired outcomes for achievement or lack of achievement.

7.9 Continually evaluates and revises the nursing care plan according to changes in the patient's health status.

MEDICAL-SURGICAL REGISTERED NURSE: PERFORMANCE EVALUATION

Name _____ Employment Date _____

Rating Period _____ To _____

Department _____ Job Title _____

Instructions Using the following rating scale, indicate the quality of performance by placing the appropriate letter on the line to the left of the item.

U*– Unsatisfactory (does not meet job requirements)
S – Satisfactory (meets job requirements)
A – Above average (exceeds job requirements)
E* – Exceptional performance

I. *Assessment:*

_____ 1. Assesses the number and level of personnel needed to provide quality patient care on the unit and collaborates with the Head Nurse or Supervisor in adjusting staffing and assignments.

_____

_____

_____ 2. Assesses the delivery of nursing care on the unit and identifies problems and any need for improvements.

_____

_____

_____ 3. Assesses the health status of assigned patients on the unit as outlined in the nursing standards.

_____

_____

3.1 Completes a comprehensive patient history and physical, including patient interview, psychological and physical assessment, as well as patient's perception of illness.

_____

_____

---

*The evaluator is expected to comment on all items rate "U" or "E."

3.2 Collects data from the patient, family and significant others, health care providers, individuals, and/or agencies in the community.

_____

_____

3.3 Collects data by: interview, observation, inspection, auscultation, palpation, and reports and records.

_____

_____

3.4 Organizes assessment data so that they are accurate, complete, and accessible, and so that they remain confidential.

_____

_____

3.5 Communicates assessment data in an orderly fashion by recording, updating, and communicating among the health team daily and by revising as appropriate.

_____

_____

II. _Planning:_

_____ 1. Serves on hospital committees and helps to review and revise policies and procedures, as directed by Head Nurse or Supervisor.

_____

_____

_____ 2. Plans and develops self-objectives.

_____

_____

_____ 3. Plans ways to solve problems and to make improvements on the unit, in collaboration with supervisory personnel.

_____

_____

_____ 4. Completes a written care plan for assigned patients on the unit. Plans the care for individual patients as well as directs and supervises others in the planning of patients' care.

_____

_____

4.1 Identifies the patient's present/potential problems from the patient assessment.

_____

_____

a. Patient's health status is determined,

_____

_____

b. Health status is compared to the norms,

_____

_____

c. Problems are given priority according to impact upon that patient's health status.

_____

_____

4.2 Formulates desired outcomes, specific to the patient problems and established norms.

_____

_____

4.3 Ensures that desired outcomes are mutually agreed upon by the patient and nurse and are: (a) specific, (b) measurable within a certain time frame, and (c) consistent with other health provider's expectations.

_____

_____

4.4 Incorporates home health care into the patient's desired outcomes. This includes but is not limited to teaching about the disease process and complications, medications, diet, exercise/activity, self-care techniques and materials, and available support systems and resources.

_____

_____

III. _Implementation:_

_____ 1. Implements activities necessary to meeting self-objectives.

_____

_____

_____ 2. Participates in implementing planned changes and activities to improve nursing service.

_____

_____

_____ 3. Holds self accountable for the delivery of quality nursing care.

_____

_____

_____ 4. Promotes harmonious relationships and favorable attitudes among the health care team.

_____

_____

_____ 5. Supports and adheres to administrative and nursing service policies and procedures.

_____

_____

_____ 6. Assists with orientation of new employees.

_____

_____

_____ 7. Acts rapidly and effectively, manages self, patients, and other employees during any emergency situation.

_____

_____

_____ 8. Attends required inservice education programs.

_____

_____

_____ 9. Formulates nursing prescriptions that delineate actions to be taken.
Prescribed actions:
9.1 Are specific to the patient's problems and the desired outcomes.

_____

_____

9.2 Are based on scientific knowledge.

_____

_____

9.3 Are based on principles of patient teaching.

_____

_____

9.4 Are based on principles of psychosocial interactions.

_____

_____

9.5 Are based on environmental factors influencing the patient's health.

_____

_____

9.6 Include human, material, and community resources.

_____

_____

9.7 Include keeping patient knowledgeable of health status and total health care plan.

_____

_____

_____ 10. Implements the actions delineated in the nursing prescriptions.
Actions implemented:
10.1 Actively involve the patient and family.

_____

_____

10.2 Are based on current scientific knowledge.

_____

_____

10.3 Are flexible and individualized for each patient.

_____

_____

10.4 Include principles of safety.

_____

_____

10.5 Include principles of infection control.

_____

_____

_____ 11. Conforms to hospital dress code.

_____

_____

_____ 12. Is rarely sick or absent from work due to health.

_____

_____

_____ 13. Is prompt and attends report.

_____

_____

IV. *Evaluation:*

_____ 1. Evaluates self-objectives, revises and formulates new objectives.

_____

_____

_____ 2. Evaluates the effectiveness of problem-solving techniques and the activities implemented to improve nursing service.

_____

_____

_____ 3. Contributes to the performance evaluation of nursing service personnel on the unit.

_____

_____

_____ 4. Participates in evaluation of RN orientation policies and procedures and recommends revisions to Supervisor or Head Nurse.

_____

_____

_____ 5. Participates in the evaluation of inservice education programs.

_____

_____

_____ 6. Evaluates achievement or lack of achievement of desired outcomes.

6.1 Data are collected concerning the patient's health status.

_____

_____

6.2 Data are compared to the specific desired outcomes.

_____

_____

6.3 Includes the patient's evaluation of the achievement of desired outcomes.

_____

_____

6.4 Reassesses nursing actions for effectiveness in achieving desired outcomes.

_____

_____

_____ 7. From evaluation of achievement or lack of achievement of desired outcomes, reassesses and revises the nursing care plan.

From evaluation:

7.1 Reassesses the patient problems.

7.2 Reassesses desired outcomes to determine if appropriate, realistic, and in correct priority.

7.3 Reassesses nursing prescriptions to determine if appropriate, realistic, and stated accurately.

From reassessment:

7.4 Determines new patient present/potential problems.

7.5 From new patient problems, formulates and revises desired outcomes.

7.6 Revises nursing prescriptions.

7.7 Implements new actions in order to carry out revised prescriptions.

7.8 Continually evaluates desired outcomes for achievement or lack of achievement.

7.9 Continually evaluates and revises the nursing care plan according to changes in the patient's health status.

MEDICAL-SURGICAL REGISTERED NURSE: SCORING PROCEDURE

Instructions: Total the number of each item and multiply times the appropriate number. Add these totals to make the score.

U _____ × 0 = _____

S _____ × 1 = _____

A _____ × 2 = _____

E _____ × 3 = _____   _____ Total Score

Compare total score to the following scale to determine rank:

U	S	A	E
0 to 23	24 to 42	43 to 64	65 to 81

Overall Performance Review Score _____.

ALL ITEMS IN THE FOLLOWING SECTION MUST BE COMPLETED:

A. Interviewer's comments on overall review _____
_____
_____

B. Additional suggestions for overall work improvement and goals for next evaluation _____
_____
_____
_____

C. Self-objectives _____
_____
_____
_____

_____
Date

_____
Date

_____
Date

_____
Employee's signature

_____
Interviewer's signature

_____
Director of Nursing

MEDICAL-SURGICAL LICENSED PRACTICAL NURSE: JOB DESCRIPTION

Position Requirements: Graduate from an accredited school for Licensed Practical Nurses with current licensure in the State of Alabama. Membership in LPN Association desired but not required. Participates in educational conferences and updates and maintains professional knowledge and skills related to areas of practice.

Position Accountable for: All nursing care behaviors described in the Medical-Surgical Licensed Practical Nurse job description.

Position Accountable to: Registered Nurse in charge of unit, Supervisor, Head Nurse, Director of Nursing, and patient and family.

Position Summary: Performs the functions of a licensed practical nurse in assessing, planning, implementing, and evaluating all assigned patient care in collaboration with an RN on a unit. Is accountable for all patient care she gives during a shift. Is responsible for adhering to all Standards of Nursing Practice, for managing supplies and equipment with the direction of the RN in charge of the unit, and for promoting teamwork with physicians and personnel of other departments.

I. *Assessment*
1. Assesses nursing care given by self and identifies problems and/or need for improvement and communicates this information to the RN in charge.
2. Assesses the health status of patients included in her assignment as outlined in the nursing standards.
   2.1 Completes those portions of the patient assessment as directed by the RN and Supervisor.
   2.2 Collects data from the patient, family and significant others, health care providers, individuals, and/or agencies in the community.
   2.3 Collects data by: interview, observation, inspection, auscultation, palpation, and reports and records.
   2.4 Organizes assessment data so that they are accurate, complete, and accessible, and so that they remain confidential.
   2.5 Communicates assessment data in an orderly fashion by recording, updating, and communicating among the health team daily and revising as appropriate.

II. *Planning*
  1. Reviews and revises policies and procedures when requested.
  2. Plans and develops self-objectives with immediate supervisor, in conjunction with performance evaluation.
  3. Suggests ways to solve problems and make improvements on the unit.
  4. In collaboration with the Registered Nurse contributes to the formulation of assigned patient's care plans, as outlined in the nursing standards.
    4.1 Identifies patient problems.
    4.2 Formulates desired outcomes.
    4.3 Communicates the above to the Registered Nurse.

III. *Implementation*
  1. Implements activities necessary to meeting self-objectives.
  2. Cooperates with the RN in implementing planned changes and activities to improve nursing care on the unit.
  3. Promotes harmonious relationships and favorable attitudes among the health care team.
  4. Supports and adheres to administrative and nursing service policies and procedures.
  5. Assists with orientation of new employees.
  6. Is knowledgeable of equipment, manages self, and assists with management of assigned patients during emergencies.
  7. Attends required inservice education programs.
  8. Participates with RN on the unit in the implementation of assigned patients' care plans.
  9. Documents nursing actions implemented and effectiveness of implementation in the nurses' notes.
  10. Conforms to hospital dress code.
  11. Is rarely sick or absent from work due to health.
  12. Is prompt and attends report.

IV. *Evaluation*
  1. Evaluates the nursing care she gives.
  2. Evaluates self-objectives and determines need for new objectives.
  3. Evaluates the effectiveness of problem-solving techniques and activities implemented to improve nursing care on the unit.
  4. Evaluates LPN orientation policies and procedures and recommends revisions.
  5. Participates in the evaluation of inservice education programs.
  6. Participates with the Registered Nurse in the evaluation and revision of assigned patient's care plans.

MEDICAL-SURGICAL LICENSED PRACTICAL NURSE: PERFORMANCE EVALUATION

Name _____ Employment Date _____

Rating Period _____ To _____

Department _____ Job Title _____

Instructions: Using the following rating scale, indicate the quality of performance by placing the appropriate letter on the line to the left of the item.

    U* – Unsatisfactory (does not meet job requirements)
    S – Satisfactory (meets job requirements)
    A – Above average (exceeds job requirements)
    E* – Expectional performance

I. *Assessment:*

_____ 1. Assesses nursing care given by self and identifies problems and/or need for improvement and communicates this information to the RN in charge.

_____

_____

_____ 2. Assesses the health status of patients included in her assignment as outlined in the nursing standards.

    2.1 Completes those portions of the patient assessment as directed by the RN and Supervisor.

_____

_____

    2.2 Collects data from the patient, family and significant others, health care providers, individuals, and/or agencies in the community.

_____

_____

    2.3 Collects data by: interview, observation, inspection, auscultation, palpation, and reports and records.

_____

_____

---

*The evaluator is expected to comment on all items rated "U" or "E."

2.4 Organizes assessment data so that they are accurate, complete, and accessible, and so that they remain confidential.

_____

_____

2.5 Communicates assessment data in an orderly fashion by recording, updating, and communicating among the health team daily and revising as appropriate.

_____

_____

II. _Planning:_

_____ 1. Reviews and revises policies and procedures when requested.

_____

_____

_____ 2. Plans and develops self-objectives with immediate supervisor, in conjunction with performance evaluation.

_____

_____

_____ 3. Suggests ways to solve problems and make improvements on the unit.

_____

_____

_____ 4. In collaboration with the Registered Nurse contributes to the formulation of assigned patient's care plans, as outlined in the nursing standards.
4.1 Identifies patient problems.

_____

_____

4.2 Formulates desired outcomes.

_____

_____

4.3 Communicates the above to the Registered Nurse.

_____

_____

III. _Implementation:_

_____ 1. Implements activities necessary to meeting self-objectives.

_____

_____

_____ 2. Cooperates with the RN in implementing planned changes and activities to improve nursing care on the unit.

_____

_____

_____ 3. Promotes harmonious relationships and favorable attitudes among the health care team.

_____

_____

_____ 4. Supports and adheres to administrative and nursing service policies and procedures.

_____

_____

_____ 5. Assists with orientation of new employees.

_____

_____

_____ 6. Is knowledgeable of equipment, manages self, and assists with management of assigned patients during emergencies.

_____

_____

_____ 7. Attends required inservice education programs.

_____

_____

_____ 8. Participates with RN on the unit in the implementation of assigned patients' care plans.

_____

_____

_____ 9. Documents nursing actions implemented and effectiveness of implementation in the nurses' notes.

_____

_____

_____ 10. Conforms to hospital dress codes.

_____

_____

_____ 11. Is rarely sick or absent from work due to health.

_____

_____

_____ 12. Is prompt and attends report.

_____

_____

IV. *Evaluation:*

_____ 1. Evaluates the nursing care she gives.

_____

_____

_____ 2. Evaluates self-objectives and determines need for new objectives.

_____

_____

_____ 3. Evaluates the effectiveness of problem-solving techniques and activities implemented to improve nursing care on the unit.

_____

_____

_____ 4. Evaluates LPN orientation policies and procedures and recommends
revisions.

_____

_____

_____ 5. Participates in the evaluation of inservice education programs.

_____

_____

_____ 6. Participates with the Registered Nurse in the evaluation and revision
of assigned patients' care plans.

_____

_____

MEDICAL-SURGICAL LICENSED PRACTICAL NURSE: SCORING PROCEDURE

Instructions: Total the number of each item and multiply times the appropriate number. Add these totals to make the score.

U _____ × 0 = _____

S _____ × 1 = _____

A _____ × 2 = _____

E _____ × 3 = _____   _____ Total Score

Compare total score to the following scale to determine rank:

U	S	A	E
0 to 21	22 to 37	38 to 57	58 to 72

Overall Performance Review Score _____.

ALL ITEMS IN THE FOLLOWING SECTION MUST BE COMPLETED:

A. Interviewer's comments on overall review _____
_____
_____

B. Additional suggestions for overall work improvement and goals for next evaluation _____
_____
_____
_____

C. Self-objectives _____
_____
_____
_____

_____   _____
Date   Employee's signature

_____   _____
Date   Interviewer's signature

_____   _____
Date   Director of Nursing

106

8

Intensive and Coronary Care Nursing Practice

STANDARDS OF INTENSIVE AND CORONARY CARE NURSING PRACTICE

STANDARD I

Assessment is the identification and gathering of data concerning the health status of the patient. This process is complete, continuous, and systematic as evidenced by:

1. *A comprehensive patient history and physical:*
   a. *Patient interview:*
   Chief complaint
   History of present illness
   Allergies
   Medications
   Past medical/surgical history
   Family history
   Cultural, environmental, and socioeconomic conditions
   Activities of daily living
   Personal habits
   Food and fluid preferences
   Appetite/weight changes
   Sleep/rest pattern interruption
   Fatigue/activity tolerance
   Available and accessible human, community, and material resources
   b. *Psychological assessment:*
   Emotional Status
   Patterns of coping
   Concerns during hospitalization
   c. *Physical assessment:*
   Personal hygiene and grooming
   Nutritional status
   Pain
   Vital signs
   Physical status
   Specific intensive and coronary care assessments:
   1. *Head, ears, eyes, nose, throat:*
      Pupil response
      Drainage
      Equilibrium
      Visual disturbances
      Hearing disturbances
      Dysphagia
      Lesions
      Sclera
   2. *Heart:*
      Apical impulse

      Heart sounds
      Heart rate and quality
      Thrills
      Palpitations
3. *Respiratory system:*
      Respiratory rate and quality
      Breath sounds
      Dyspnea
      Exceptional dypsnea
      Orthopnea
      Cough
      Sputum
      Chest symmetry
      Nausea
      Retractions
4. *Vascular system:*
      Bruits
      Neck veins
      Peripheral pulses
      Peripheral edema
5. *Skin:*
      Color
      Moisture level
      Temperature
      Nail beds
      Turgor
      Petechiae
6. *Gastrointestinal:*
      Nausea/vomiting
      Diarrhea/constipation
      Bowel sounds
      Distention
      Masses
      Ascites
7. *Musculoskeletal system:*
      Muscle weakness
      Muscle impairment
      Range of motion
8. *Mental/neurological:*
      Level of consciousness
      Mental status
      Seizure activity
      Syncope
9. *Genitourinary system:*
      Frequency
      Hematuria
      Urinary output
      Burning
      Retention
      Nocturia

Dysuria
Incontinence

d. *Perception of illness:*
Understanding of disease process/illness
Understanding of reasons for hospitalization
Desired outcome from hospitalization

2. *The collection of data from available sources:*
Patient, family, significant other
Health care providers
Individuals and/or agencies in the community

3. *The collection of data by scientific methodology:*
Interview
Observation
Inspection
Auscultation
Palpation

4. *The collection of data by continuous interpretation/assessment of reports and records:*
EKG
Radiology studies
Hematology studies
Chemistry studies
Coagulation studies
Urinalysis
Serial cardiac enzymes
Previous records
Arterial blood gases

5. *The organization of data in a systematic arrangement:*
The arrangement provides:
a. Accurate collection
b. Complete collection
c. Accessibility
d. Confidentiality

6. *The communication of data in an orderly fashion:*
Data are recorded for each shift, daily.
Data are updated by each shift, daily.
Data are revised and recorded as appropriate.
Data are communicated verbally among health team, daily.

STANDARD II

Nursing care planning consists of determining patient problems and desired outcomes. Planning involves preparing the patient for home care. This is evidenced by:

1. *The identification of present/potential patient problems, from the patient assessment:*
Data are grouped into meaningful arrangement, based upon scientific knowledge.
Patient's health status is determined.

Patient's health status is compared to the norms.

Present and potential problems are identified.

Problems are given priority according to impact upon patient's health status.

2. *The formulation of desired outcomes:*

Patient (family, significant other) and nurse mutually agree upon the patient's present/potential health problems.

Patient and nurse mutually agree upon desired outcomes.

Desired outcomes are congruent with the patient problems and established norms.

Desired outcomes are specific.

Desired outcomes are measurable within a certain time frame.

Desired outcomes are consistent with other health providers' expectations.

Desired outcomes are established to restore patient's optimal functioning capabilities.

3. *The incorporation of home health care into desired outcomes:*

Providing support systems, health information and resources that will enable the patient to identify and accept necessary modifications in life-style.

Patient/family demonstration of knowledge of therapeutic regimen:

a. Disease process and complications

b. Medication

c. Diet

d. Exercise/activity pattern

e. Self-care techniques and materials

f. Available support systems and resources

STANDARD III

The plan of care is implemented in order to achieve the desired outcome. This is evidenced by:

1. *The formulation of nursing prescriptions that delineate actions to be taken: Prescribed actions:*

Are specific to identified patient problems and desired outcomes.

Are based on current scientific knowledge.

Incorporate principles of patient teaching.

Incorporate principles of psychosocial interactions.

Incorporate environmental factors influencing the patient's health.

Include human, material, and community resources.

Include keeping patient knowledgeable of health status and total health care plan.

2. *The implementation of actions delineated in the nursing prescriptions: Actions implemented:*

Actively involve the patient and family.

Are consistent with the nursing prescriptions.

Are based upon current scientific knowledge.

Are flexible and individualized for each patient.

Include principles of safety.

Include principles of infection control.

STANDARD IV

Outcomes of Nursing Actions are evaluated for further assessment and planning. This is evidenced by:

1. *Evaluating the achievement of desired outcomes:*
   Data are collected concerning the patient's health status.
   Data are compared to the specific desired outcomes.
   The patient and nurse evaluate the achievement of desired outcomes.
2. *Reassessment of the nursing care plan:*
   Outcome of nursing actions direct the reassessment of identified patient problems.
   Outcome of nursing actions direct assessment of desired outcomes (assess the desired outcome to determine if appropriate, realistic, and in correct priority).
   Outcome of nursing action direct reassessment of nursing prescriptions (assess the nursing prescriptions to determine if appropriate, realistic, and stated accurately). Nursing actions are assessed for effectiveness in achieving desired outcomes.
3. *Further planning as directed by the reassessment:*
   Determines new patient present/potential problems.
   The formulation and revision of desired outcomes.
   Revised desired outcomes direct the revising of nursing prescriptions.
   Revised prescriptions direct new actions to be implemented toward desired outcomes.
   Desired outcomes are continually evaluated for achievement.
   The plan of care is continually evaluated and revised according to changes in the patient's health status.

INTENSIVE AND CORONARY CARE SUPERVISOR: JOB DESCRIPTION

Position Requirements:	Graduate from an accredited school of nursing with current licensure as a registered nurse in the State of Alabama. At least 3 years clinical experience in Intensive Coronary Care with 1 year of supervisory training.
Professional Requirements:	Pursues programs of continuing education consistent with requirements of the Alabama Nurses' Association. Participates in educational conferences and updates and maintains professional knowledge and skills related to the management areas of responsibility.
Position Accountable for:	All nursing care behaviors described in the Intensive and Coronary Care Unit Supervisor job description.
Position Accountable to:	Director of Nursing Service.
Position Summary:	Performs the primary functions of a professional nurse leader in assessing, planning, directing, implementing, and evaluating patient care in Intensive and Coronary Care Unit on a 24-hour basis. Is responsible for ensuring continuity of care with other shifts. Is responsible for meeting the Joint Commission Standards of Intensive and Coronary Care, for managing all assigned personnel, supplies, and equipment in the unit, and for promoting teamwork with physicians and personnel of other departments.

I. *Assessment*
1. Assesses the number and level of personnel needed to provide quality patient care and adjusts staffing and assignments appropriately.
2. Assesses the delivery of nursing care and identifies problems and any need for improvements.
3. Ensures that the health status of patients in the unit is assessed on a daily basis as outlined in nursing standards:
   3.1 A comprehensive patient history and physical including patient interview, psychological and physical assessment, as well as patient's perception of illness is completed on each patient.
   3.2 Data are collected from patient, family, significant others, health care providers, and individuals and/or agencies in the community.

3.3 Data are collected by: interview, observation, inspection, auscultation, and palpation.

3.4 The assessment and interpretation of reports and records includes:

EKG	Urinalysis
Radiology Studies	Serial Cardiac Enzymes
Hematology Studies	Previous Records
Chemistry Studies	Arterial Blood Gases
Coagulation Studies	

3.5 The recognition and assessment of initial/slight alterations in the patient's body systems (i.e., heart and lung sounds) and verbalizes this among members of the health team.

3.6 Heart patterns are interpreted, changes assessed, and pertinent information is verbalized among health team members.

3.7 Ensures the organization of assessment data so they are accurate, complete, and accessible, and so they remain confidential.

3.8 Assessment data are communicated in an orderly fashion by reporting, revising, verbalizing pertinent information among members of the health care team, and recording.

II. *Planning*

1. Serves on hospital committees.

2. Develops, reviews, and revises policies and procedures for the Intensive and Coronary Care Unit with approval of Director of Nursing.

3. Plans ways to solve problems and to make improvements in the delivery of patient care in collaboration with the Director of Nursing.

4. Ensures that all patients have a nursing care plan. Establishes individual patients' care plans as well as directs and supervises others in the formulation of patient care plans. Ensures that:

4.1 The patient's present/potential problems are identified from the patient assessment.
   a. patient's health status is determined,
   b. health status is compared to the norms,
   c. Problems are given priority according to impact on the patient's health status.

4.2 Desired outcomes are formulated specific to the patient and family's problems/needs and established norms.

4.3 Identified problems and desired outcomes are mutually agreed upon by patient, family (when appropriate), and nurse.

4.4 Desired outcomes are: (a) specific, (b) measureable within a certain time frame, and (c) consistent with other health providers' expectations.

4.5 Home health care is incorporated into desired outcomes.
   a. Support systems, health information, and resources are provided to assist the acceptance of life-style modifications.
   b. Ensures that desired outcomes include but are not limited to teaching: disease process and complications, medication, diet, exercise/activity pattern, self-care techniques and materials, and available support systems and resources.

III. *Implementation*
1. Implements activities necessary to meeting self-objectives.
2. Promotes the achievement of Intensive Coronary Care Unit objectives.
3. Directs, supervises, and participates in implementing planned changes and activities to improve the department in collaboration with the Director of Nursing.
4. Ensures that Intensive and Coronary Care Standards of Nursing Care are implemented and assists in monitoring of standards as necessary.
5. Holds self and staff accountable for the delivery of quality nursing care.
6. Acts rapidly and effectively, follows hospital policies and procedures, and utilizes principles of management in any emergency situation.
7. Promotes harmonious relationships and favorable attitudes among the health care team.
8. Interprets, supports, and recommends administrative, nursing service, and department policies and procedures for employees. Applies knowledge and skills of management.
9. Directs and assists with orientation of new employees.
10. Keeps the Director of Nursing informed on reportable situations and nursing unit needs.
11. Attends required inservice education programs.
12. Ensures that nursing prescriptions are formulated as outlined in the nursing standards that delineate actions to be taken. Ensures that:
    12.1 Prescribed actions are specific to patient problems and desired outcomes.
    12.2 Prescribed actions are based on current scientific knowledge.
    12.3 Principles of patient teaching are incorporated into the prescribed actions.
    12.4 Principles of psychosocial interactions are incorporated into the prescribed actions.
    12.5 Environmental factors influencing the patient's health are incorporated into the prescribed actions.
    12.6 Prescribed actions include human, material, and community resources.
    12.7 Prescribed actions include keeping patient knowledgeable of health status and total health care plan.
13. Ensures that the actions delineated in the nursing prescriptions are implemented. Actions implemented:
    13.1 Actively involve the patient and family.
    13.2 Are consistent with nursing prescriptions.
    13.3 Are based on current scientific knowledge.
    13.4 Are flexible and individualized for each patient.
    13.5 Include principles of safety.
    13.6 Include principles of infection control.
14. Serves as consultant in technical and professional matters for personnel.

15. Participates and contributes to a unified Quality Assurance Program.

16. Participates in the provision of inservice education programs related to Intensive and Coronary Nursing Care.

17. Ensures that an RN from the unit responds immediately to a Code "9" (Cardiac Arrest) and effectively takes charge and initiates necessary treatment until a physician arrives.

18. Ensures personnel demonstrate knowledge of location, care, and operation of Intensive Care Unit equipment. This includes but is not limited to: monitors, defibrillation equipment, crash carts and contents, trays (trachea, cvp), pacemaker, and ventilator.

19. Ensures Intensive Coronary Care Unit is clean, organized, and stocked with necessary supplies.

20. Ensures the Intensive Coronary Care Unit provides a calm, reassuring atmosphere and provides for effective communication with each patient's family to reduce stress.

21. Is rarely sick or absent from work due to health.

22. Conforms to hospital dress code.

23. Is prompt and attends report.

IV. *Evaluation*

1. Continually evaluates the Standards of Intensive and Coronary Care Nursing Practice by reviewing nursing care plans, assessing patients, reviewing charts, interviewing, observing, participating in quality assurance activities, and employing other means of evaluation. Revises standards as appropriate.

2. Evaluates policies and procedures and revises as necessary in collaboration with Director of Nursing.

3. Evaluates self-objectives and determines need for revision and new objectives.

4. Evaluates the effectiveness of problem-solving techniques and activities implemented to improve the unit.

5. Evaluates the performance of nursing service personnel.

6. Evaluates the achievement of Intensive Coronary Care nursing service objectives.

7. Evaluates emergencies and any hospital disaster and recommends revisions in policies and procedures and/or need for improvement in employee performance.

8. Evaluates orientation policies and procedures and recommends revisions as necessary.

9. Evaluates inservice education programs.

10. Ensures that desired outcomes are evaluated for achievement or lack of achievement.
    10.1 Data are collected concerning the patient's health status.
    10.2 Data are compared to the specific desired outcomes.
    10.3 The patient and nurse evaluate the achievement of desired outcomes.

11. Ensures that the nursing care plans are reassessed and revised according to the evaluation of achievement or lack of achievement of desired outcomes.

From evaluation:

11.1 Reassesses the patient problems.

11.2 Reassesses desired outcomes to determine if appropriate, realistic, and in correct priority.

11.3 Reassesses nursing prescriptions to determine if appropriate, realistic, and stated accurately.

11.4 Reassesses nursing actions for effectiveness in achieving desired outcomes.

From reassessment:

11.5 New patient present/potential problems are determined.

11.6 From new patient problems desired outcomes are formulated and revised.

11.7 Nursing prescriptions are revised.

11.8 New actions are implemented in order to carry out revised prescriptions.

11.9 Desired outcomes are continually evaluated for achievement or lack of achievement.

11.10 The nursing care plan is continually evaluated and revised according to changes in the patient's health status.

INTENSIVE AND CORONARY CARE
SUPERVISOR: PERFORMANCE EVALUATION

Name _____ Employment Date _____

Rating Period _____ To _____

Department _____ Job Title _____

Instructions: Using the following rating scale, indicate the quality of performance by placing the appropriate letter on the line to the left of the item.

U* – Unsatisfactory (does not meet job requirements)
S – Satisfactory (meets job requirements)
A – Above average (exceeds job requirements)
E* – Exceptional performance

I. *Assessment:*

_____ 1. Assesses the number and level of personnel needed to provide quality patient care and adjusts staffing and assignments appropriately.

_____

_____

_____ 2. Assesses the delivery of nursing care and identifies problems and any need for improvements.

_____

_____

_____ 3. Ensures that the health status of patients in the unit is assessed on a daily basis as outlined in nursing standards:
    3.1 A comprehensive patient history and physical, including patient interview, psychological and physical assessment, as well as patient's perception of illness is completed on each patient.

_____

    3.2 Data are collected from patient, family, significant others, health care providers, and individuals and/or agencies in the community.

_____

_____

_____

*The evaluator is expected to comment on all items rated "U" or "E."

118

3.3 Data are collected by interview, observation, inspection, auscultation and palpation.

_____

_____

3.4 The assessment and interpretation of reports and records includes:

EKG	Urinalysis
Radiology studies	Serial cardiac enzymes
Hematology studies	Previous records
Chemistry studies	Arterial blood gases
Coagulation studies	

_____

3.5 The recognition and assessment of initial/slight alterations in the
patient's body systems (i.e., heart and lung sounds) and verbalizes this among members of the health team.

_____

3.6 Heart patterns are interpreted, changes assessed, and pertinent
information is verbalized among health team members.

_____

3.7 Ensures the organization of assessment data so they are accurate, complete, and accessible, and so they remain confidential.

_____

3.8 Assessment data are communicated in an orderly fashion by
reporting, revising, verbalizing pertinent information among
members of the health care team, and recording.

_____

_____

II. _Planning:_

_____ 1. Serves on hospital committees.

_____

_____

_____ 2. Develops, reviews, and revises policies and procedures for the Intensive and Coronary Care Unit with approval of Director of Nursing.

_____

_____

_____ 3. Plans ways to solve problems and to make improvements in the delivery of patient care in collaboration with the Director of Nursing.

_____

_____

_____ 4. Ensures that all patients have a nursing care plan. Establishes individual patient's care plans as well as directs and supervises others in the formulation of patient care plans. Ensures that:

4.1 The patient's present/potential problems are identified from the patient assessment.
   a. patient's health status is determined,
   b. health status is compared to the norms,
   c. problems are given priority according to impact on the patient's health status.

_____

_____

4.2 Desired outcomes are formulated specific to the patient and family's problems/needs and established norms.

_____

_____

4.3 Identified problems and desired outcomes are mutually agreed upon by patient, family (when appropriate), and nurse.

_____

_____

4.4 Desired outcomes are: (a) specific, (b) measurable within a certain time frame, and (c) consistent with other health providers' expectations.

_____

_____

4.5 Home health care is incorporated into desired outcomes:
   a. Support systems, health information, and resources are provided to assist the acceptance of life-style modifications,
   b. Ensures that desired outcomes include but are not limited to teaching: disease process and complications, medication, diet, exercise/activity patterns, self-care techniques and materials, and available support systems and resources.

_____

_____

III. *Implementation:*

_____ 1. Implements activities necessary to meeting self-objectives.

_____

_____

_____ 2. Promotes the achievement of Intensive Coronary Care Unit objectives.

_____

_____

_____ 3. Directs, supervises, and participates in implementing planned changes and activities to improve the department in collaboration with the Director of Nursing.

_____

_____

_____ 4. Ensures that Intensive and Coronary Care Standards of Nursing Care are implemented, assists in monitoring of standards as necessary.

_____

_____

_____ 5. Holds self and staff accountable for the delivery of quality nursing care.

_____

_____

_____ 6. Acts rapidly and effectively, follows hospital policies and procedures, and utilizes principles of management in any emergency situation.

_____

_____

_____ 7. Promotes harmonious relationships and favorable attitudes among the health care team.

_____

_____

_____ 8. Interprets, supports, and recommends administrative, nursing service, and department policies and procedures for employees. Applies knowledge and skills of management.

_____

_____

_____ 9. Directs and assists with orientation of new employees.

_____

_____

_____ 10. Keeps the Director of Nursing informed on reportable situations and nursing unit needs.

_____

_____

_____ 11. Attends required inservice education programs.

_____

_____

_____ 12. Ensures that nursing prescriptions are formulated as outlined in the nursing standards that delineate actions to be taken. Ensures that:

12.1 Prescribed actions are specific to patient problems and desired outcomes.

_____

12.2 Prescribed actions are based on current scientific knowledge.

_____

12.3 Principles of patient teaching are incorporated into the prescribed actions.

_____

12.4 Principles of psychosocial interactions are incorporated into the prescribed actions.

_____

12.5 Environmental factors influencing the patient's health are incorporated into the prescribed actions.

_____

12.6 Prescribed actions include human, material, and community resources.

_____

12.7 Prescribed actions include keeping patient knowledgeable of health status and total health care plan.

_____

_____

_____ 13. Ensures that the actions delineated in the nursing prescriptions are implemented. Actions implemented:

13.1 Actively involve the patient and family.

_____

_____

13.2 Are consistent with nursing prescriptions.

_____

_____

13.3 Are based on current scientific knowledge.

_____

_____

13.4 Are flexible and individualized for each patient.

_____

_____

13.5 Include principles of safety.

_____

_____

13.6 Include principles of infection control.

_____

_____

_____ 14. Serves as consultant in technical and professional matters for personnel.

_____

_____

_____ 15. Participates and contributes to a unified Quality Assurance Program.

_____

_____

_____ 16. Participates in the provision of inservice education programs related to Intensive and Coronary Nursing Care.

_____

_____

_____ 17. Ensures that an RN from the unit responds immediately to a Code "9" (cardiac arrest) and effectively takes charge and initiates necessary treatment until a physician arrives.

_____

_____

_____ 18. Ensures personnel demonstrate knowledge of location, care, and operation of Intensive Care Unit equipment. This includes but is not limited to: monitors, defibrillation equipment, crash carts and contents, trays (trachea, cvp), pacemaker, and ventilator.

_____

_____

_____ 19. Ensures Intensive Coronary Care Unit is clean, organized, and stocked with necessary supplies.

_____

_____

_____ 20. Ensures the Intensive Coronary Care Unit provides a calm, reassuring atmosphere and provides for effective communication with each patient's family to reduce stress.

_____

_____

_____ 21. Is rarely sick or absent from work due to health.

_____

_____

_____ 22. Conforms to hospital dress code.

_____

_____

_____ 23. Is prompt and attends report.

_____

_____

IV. _Evaluation:_

_____ 1. Continually evaluates the Standards of Intensive and Coronary Care Nursing Practice by reviewing nursing care plans, assessing patients, reviewing charts, interviewing, observing, participating in quality assurance activities, and employing other means of evaluation. Revises standards as appropriate.

_____

_____

_____ 2. Evaluates policies and procedures and revises as necessary in collaboration with Director of Nursing.

_____

_____

_____ 3. Evaluates self-objectives and determines need for revision and new objectives.

_____

_____

_____ 4. Evaluates the effectiveness of problem-solving techniques and activities implemented to improve the unit.

_____

_____

_____ 5. Evaluates the performance of nursing service personnel.

_____

_____

_____ 6. Evaluates the achievement of Intensive Coronary Care nursing service objectives.

_____

_____

_____ 7. Evaluates emergencies and any hospital disaster and recommends revisions in policies and procedures and/or need for improvement in employee performance.

_____

_____

_____ 8. Evaluates orientation policies and procedures and recommends revisions as necessary.

_____

_____

_____ 9. Evaluates inservice education programs.

_____

_____

_____ 10. Ensures that desired outcomes are evaluated for achievement or lack of achievement.
    10.1 Data are collected concerning the patient's health status.

_____

_____

    10.2 Data are compared to the specific desired outcomes.

_____

_____

    10.3 The patient and nurse evaluate the achievement of desired outcomes.

_____

_____

_____ 11. Ensures that the nursing care plans are reassessed and revised according to the evaluation of achievement or lack of achievement of desired outcomes.
    From evaluation:
    11.1   Reassesses the patient problems.

_____

_____

11.2 Reassesses desired outcomes to determine if appropriate, realistic, and in correct priority.

___

11.3 Reassesses nursing prescriptions to determine if appropriate, realistic, and stated accurately.

___

11.4 Reassesses nursing actions for effectiveness in achieving desired outcomes.

___

From reassessment:

11.5 New patient present/potential problems are determined.

___

11.6 From new patient problems desired outcomes are formulated and revised.

___

11.7 Nursing prescriptions are revised.

___

11.8 New actions are implemented in order to carry out revised prescriptions.

___

11.9 Desired outcomes are continually evaluated for achievement or lack of achievement.

___

11.10 The nursing care plan is continually evaluated and revised according to changes in the patient's health status.

___

INTENSIVE AND CORONARY CARE
SUPERVISOR: SCORING PROCEDURE

Instructions: Total the number of each item and multiply times the appropriate number. Add these totals to make the score.

$$U \underline{\hspace{2cm}} \times 0 = \underline{\hspace{2cm}}$$

$$S \underline{\hspace{2cm}} \times 1 = \underline{\hspace{2cm}}$$

$$A \underline{\hspace{2cm}} \times 2 = \underline{\hspace{2cm}}$$

$$E \underline{\hspace{2cm}} \times 3 = \underline{\hspace{2cm}} \qquad \underline{\hspace{2cm}} \text{ Total Score}$$

Compare total score to the following scale to determine rank:

U	S	A	E
0 to 36	37 to 65	66 to 97	98 to 123

Overall Performance Review Score _____.

ALL ITEMS IN THE FOLLOWING SECTION MUST BE COMPLETED:

A. Interviewer's comments on overall review _____

_____

_____

B. Additional suggestions for overall work improvement and goals for next evaluation _____

_____

_____

C. Self-objectives _____

_____

_____

_____

Date _____   Employee's signature _____

Date _____   Interviewer's signature _____

Date _____   Director of Nursing _____

INTENSIVE AND CORONARY CARE REGISTERED NURSE: JOB DESCRIPTION

Position Requirements: Graduate from an accredited school of nursing with current licensure as a registered nurse in the State of Alabama. Specific orientation for Intensive Coronary Care Nursing.

Professional Requirements: Pursues programs of continuing education consistent with requirements of the Alabama Nurses' Association. Participates in educational conferences and updates and maintains professional knowledge and skills related to areas of responsibility.

Position Accountable for: All nursing care behaviors described in the Intensive and Coronary Care Registered Nurse job description.

Position Accountable to: Intensive and Coronary Care Unit Supervisor, Director of Nursing, the patient and family.

Position Summary: Performs the primary functions of an RN in assessing, planning, implementing, and evaluating the care of all patients in the unit during her shift. Is responsible for meeting the established standards of Intensive Coronary Nursing Practice, for managing all assigned personnel, supplies, and equipment in the unit, and for promoting teamwork with physicians and personnel of other departments.

I. *Assessment*
1. Assesses the number and level of personnel needed to provide quality patient care in the unit and collaborates with the Supervisor in adjusting staffing and assignments.
2. Assesses the delivery of nursing care in the unit and identifies problems and any need for improvements.
3. Assesses the health care status of all assigned patients in the unit as outlined in the nursing standards.
   3.1 Completes a comprehensive patient history and physical including patient interview, psychological and physical assessment, as well as patient's perception of illness.
   3.2 Collects data from patient, family, significant others, health care providers, and individuals and/or agencies in the community.
   3.3 Collects data by interview, observation, inspection, auscultation, and palpation.

   3.4 Assesses and interprets reports and records:

EKG	Urinalysis
Radiology Studies	Serial Cardiac Enzymes
Hematology Studies	Previous Records
Chemistry Studies	Arterial Blood Gases
Coagulation Studies	

   3.5 Recognizes and assesses initial/slight alterations in the patient's body systems (i.e., heart and lung sounds) and verbalizes this among members of the health team.

   3.6 Interprets heart patterns on monitor and assesses changes in pattern, verbalizing this among members of the health team.

   3.7 Organizes assessment data so they are accurate, complete, and accessible, and so they remain confidential.

   3.8 Communicates assessment data in an orderly fashion by reporting, revising, verbalizing pertinent information among members of the health team, and recording.

II. *Planning*

   1. Serves on hospital committees and helps to review and revise policies and procedures, as directed by the Supervisor.

   2. Plans and develops self-objectives.

   3. Plans ways to solve problems and to make improvements in the unit, in collaboration with the Supervisor.

   4. Completes a written nursing care plan for all assigned patients in the unit.

      4.1 Identifies the patient's present/potential problems from the patient assessment.

         a. patient's health status is determined,

         b. health status is compared to the norms,

         c. problems are given priority according to impact upon the patient's health status.

      4.2 Formulates desired outcomes specific to the patient problems/needs and established norms.

      4.3 Ensures that desired outcomes are mutually agreed upon by the patient, family (when appropriate), and nurse.

      4.4 Formulates desired outcomes that are specific, measureable within a certain time frame, and consistent with other health providers' expectations.

      4.5 Incorporates home health care into desired outcomes:

         a. Provides support systems, health information, and resources to assist the acceptance of life-style modifications.

         b. Patient teaching including but not limited to: disease process and complications, medication, diet, exercise/activity pattern, self-care techniques and materials, and available support systems and resources.

III. *Implementation*

   1. Implements activities necessary to meeting self-objectives.

   2. Participates in implementing planned changes and activities to improve nursing service.

3. Participates in activities promoting the achievement of Intensive and Coronary Care nursing objectives.

4. Holds self and staff accountable for the delivery of quality nursing care.

5. Promotes harmonious relationships and favorable attitudes among the health care team.

6. Supports and adheres to administrative and nursing service policies and procedures.

7. Assists with orientation of new employees.

8. Acts rapidly and effectively, manages self, patients, and other employees during any emergency situation.

9. Attends required inservice education programs.

10. Formulates nursing prescriptions that delineate actions to be taken. Prescribed actions:
    10.1 Are specific to patient problem and expected outcomes.
    10.2 Are based on current scientific knowledge.
    10.3 Are based on principles of patient teaching as appropriate.
    10.4 Are based on principles of psychosocial interactions as appropriate.
    10.5 Are based on environmental factors influencing the patient's health as appropriate.
    10.6 Include human, material, and community resources.
    10.7 Include keeping patient knowledgeable of health status and total health care plan.

11. Implements the actions delineated in the nursing prescriptions. Actions implemented:
    11.1 Actively involve the patient and family.
    11.2 Are consistent with nursing prescriptions.
    11.3 Are based on current scientific knowledge.
    11.4 Are flexible and individualized for each patient.
    11.5 Include principles of safety.
    11.6 Include principles of infection control.

12. Responds immediately to a Code "9" (cardiac arrest) and effectively takes charge and initiates necessary treatment until a physician arrives.

13. Is knowledgeable of location, care, and operation of Intensive Care Unit equipment. This includes but is not limited to: monitors, defibrillation equipment, crash carts and contents, trays (trachea, CVP), pacemaker, and ventilator.

14. Maintains clean, organized unit and restocks supplies as necessary.

15. Provides a calm, reassuring atmosphere and communicates effectively with each patient's family to reduce stress.

16. Conforms to hospital dress code.

17. Is rarely sick or absent from work due to health.

18. Is prompt and attends report.

IV. *Evaluation*
1. Evaluates self-objectives.
2. Evaluates the effectiveness of problem-solving techniques and the activities implemented to improve the unit.
3. Contributes to the performance evaluation of nursing service personnel in the unit.
4. Participates in the evaluation of RN orientation policies and procedures and recommends revisions to the Supervisor.
5. Participates in the evaluation of inservice education programs.
6. Evaluates achievement or lack of achievement of desired outcomes.
   6.1 Data are collected concerning the patient's health status.
   6.2 Data are compared to the specific desired outcomes.
   6.3 Includes the patient in evaluation of the achievement of desired outcomes.
7. From evaluation of achievement or lack of achievement of desired outcomes, reassesses and revises the nursing care plan.
   From evaluation:
   7.1 Reassesses the patient problems.
   7.2 Reassesses desired outcomes and determines if appropriate, realistic, and in correct priority.
   7.3 Reassesses nursing prescriptions to determine if appropriate, realistic, and stated accurately.
   7.4 Reassesses nursing actions for effectiveness in achieving desired outcomes.

   From reassessment:
   7.5 Determines new patient present/potential problems.
   7.6 From new patient problems, formulates and revises desired outcomes.
   7.7 Revises nursing prescriptions.
   7.8 Implements new actions in order to carry out revised prescriptions.
   7.9 Continually evaluates desired outcomes for achievement or lack of achievement.
   7.10 Continually evaluates and revises the nursing care plan according to changes in the patient's health status.

INTENSIVE AND CORONARY CARE REGISTERED NURSE: PERFORMANCE EVALUATION

Name _____ Employment Date _____

Rating Period _____ To _____

Department _____ Job Title _____

Instructions: Using the following rating scale, indicate the quality of performance by placing the appropriate letter on the line to the left of the item.

U* – Unsatisfactory (does not meet job requirements)
S – Satisfactory (meets job requirements)
A – Above average (exceeds job requirements)
E* – Exceptional performance

I. *Assessment:*

_____ 1. Assesses the number and level of personnel needed to provide quality patient care in the unit and collaborates with the Supervisor in adjusting staffing and assignments.

_____ 2. Assesses the delivery of nursing care in the unit and identifies any problems and any need for improvements.

_____ 3. Assesses the health care status of all assigned patients in the unit as outlined in the nursing standards.

3.1 Completes a comprehensive patient history and physical, including patient interview, psychological and physical assessment, as well as patient's perception of illness.

3.2 Collects data from patient, family, significant others, health care providers, and individuals and/or agencies in the community.

_____

*The evaluator is expected to comment on all items rated "U" or "E."

3.3 Collects data by interview, observation, inspection, auscultation, and palpation.

_____

_____

3.4 Assesses and interprets reports and records:
   EKG   Urinalysis
   Radiology studies   Serial cardiac enzymes
   Hematology studies   Previous records
   Chemistry studies   Arterial blood gases
   Coagulation studies

_____

_____

3.5 Recognizes and assesses initial/slight alterations in the patient's body systems (i.e., heart and lung sounds) and verbalizes this among members of health team.

_____

_____

3.6 Interprets heart patterns on monitor and assesses changes in pattern, verbalizing this among members of the health team.

_____

_____

3.7 Organizes assessment data so they are accurate, complete, and accessible, and so they remain confidential.

_____

_____

3.8 Communicates assessment data in an orderly fashion by reporting, revising, verbalizing pertinent information among members of the health team, and recording.

_____

_____

II. _Planning:_

_____ 1. Serves on hospital committees and helps review and revise policies and procedures, as directed by Supervisor.

_____

_____

_____ 2. Plans and develops self-objectives.

_____

_____

_____ 3. Plans ways to solve problems and to make improvements in the unit, in collaboration with the Supervisor.

_____

_____

_____ 4. Completes a written nursing care plan for all assigned patients in the unit.
   4.1 Identifies the patient's present/potential problems from the patient assessment:
      a. patient's health status is determined,
      b. health status is compared to the norms,
      c. problems are given priority according to impact upon the patient's health status.

_____

_____

   4.2 Formulates desired outcomes specific to the patient problems/ needs and established norms.

_____

_____

   4.3 Ensures that desired outcomes are mutually agreed upon by the patient, family (when appropriate), and nurse.

_____

_____

   4.4 Formulates desired outcomes so that they are specific, measurable within a certain time frame, and consistent with other health providers' expectations.

_____

_____

   4.5 Incorporates home health care into desired outcomes:
      a. Provides support systems, health information, and resources to assist the acceptance of life-style modifications,
      b. Patient teaching, including but not limited to: disease process and complications, medication, diet, exercise/activity pattern, self-care techniques and materials, and available support systems and resources.

_____

_____

III. *Implementation:*
_____ 1. Implements activities necessary to meeting self-objectives.

_____

_____

_____ 2. Participates in implementing planned changes and activities to improve nursing service.

_____

_____

_____ 3. Participates in activities promoting the achievement of Intensive and Coronary Care nursing objectives.

_____

_____

_____ 4. Holds self and staff accountable for the delivery of quality nursing care.

_____

_____

_____ 5. Promotes harmonious relationships and favorable attitudes among the health care team.

_____

_____

_____ 6. Supports and adheres to administrative and nursing service policies and procedures.

_____

_____

_____ 7. Assists with orientation of new employees.

_____

_____

_____ 8. Acts rapidly and effectively, manages self, patients, and other employees during any emergency situation.

_____

_____

_____ 9. Attends required inservice education programs.

_____

_____

_____ 10. Formulates nursing prescriptions that delineate actions to be taken.
Prescribed actions:
10.1 Are specific to patient problems and expected outcomes.

_____

_____

10.2 Are based on current scientific knowledge.

_____

_____

10.3 Are based on principles of patient teaching as appropriate.

_____

_____

10.4 Are based on principles of psychosocial interactions as appropriate.

_____

_____

10.5 Are based on environmental factors influencing the patient's health as appropriate.

_____

_____

10.6 Include human, material, and community resources.

_____

_____

10.7 Include keeping patient knowledgeable of health status and total health care plan.

_____

_____

_____ 11. Implements the actions delineated in the nursing prescriptions. Actions implemented:
11.1 Actively involve the patient and family.

_____

_____

11.2 Are consistent with nursing prescriptions.

_____

_____

11.3 Are based on current scientific knowledge.

_____

_____

11.4 Are flexible and individualized for each patient.

_____

_____

11.5 Include principles of safety.

_____

_____

11.6 Include principles of infection control.

_____

_____

_____ 12. Responds immediately to a Code "9" (cardiac arrest) and effectively takes charge and initiates necessary emergency treatment until a physician arrives.

_____

_____

_____ 13. Is knowledgeable of location, care, and operation of Intensive Care Unit equipment. This includes but is not limited to: monitors, defibrillation equipment, crash carts and contents, trays (trachea, CVP), pacemaker, and ventilator.

_____

_____

_____ 14. Maintains clean, organized unit and restocks supplies as necessary.

_____

_____

_____ 15. Provides a calm, reassuring atmosphere and communicates effectively with each patient's family to reduce stress.

_____

_____

_____ 16. Conforms to hospital dress code.

_____

_____

_____ 17. Is rarely sick or absent from work due to health.

_____

_____

_____ 18. Is prompt and attends report.

_____

_____

IV. _Evaluation:_

_____ 1. Evaluates self-objectives.

_____

_____

_____ 2. Evaluates the effectiveness of problem-solving techniques and the activities implemented to improve the unit.

_____

_____

_____ 3. Contributes to the performance evaluation of nursing service personnel in the unit.

_____

_____

_____ 4. Participates in the evaluation of RN orientation policies and procedures and recommends revisions to the Supervisor.

_____

_____

_____ 5. Participates in the evaluation of inservice education programs.

_____

_____

_____ 6. Evaluates achievement or lack of achievement of desired outcomes:
6.1 Data are collected concerning the patient's health status.

_____

6.2 Data are compared to the specific desired outcomes.

_____

6.3 Includes the patient in evaluation of the achievement of desired outcomes.

_____

_____

_____ 7. From evaluation of achievement or lack of achievement of desired outcomes, reassesses and revises the nursing care plan.
From evaluation:
7.1   Reassesses the patient problems.

_____

7.2   Reassesses desired outcomes and determines if appropriate, realistic, and in correct priority.

_____

7.3   Reassesses nursing prescriptions to determine if appropriate, realistic, and stated accurately.

_____

_____

7.4 Reassesses nursing actions for effectiveness in achieving desired outcomes.

_____

_____

From reassessment:
7.5 Determines new patient present/potential problems.

_____

_____

7.6 From new patient problems, formulates and revises desired outcomes.

_____

_____

7.7 Revises nursing prescriptions.

_____

_____

7.8 Implements new actions in order to carry out revised prescriptions.

_____

_____

7.9 Continually evaluates desired outcomes for achievement or lack of achievement.

_____

_____

7.10 Continually evaluates and revises the nursing care plan according to changes in the patient's health status.

_____

_____

INTENSIVE AND CORONARY CARE REGISTERED NURSE: SCORING PROCEDURE

Instructions: Total the number of each item and multiply times the appropriate number. Add these totals to make the score.

U _____ ×0=_____

S _____ ×1=_____

A _____ ×2=_____

E _____ ×3=_____   _____ Total Score

Compare total score to the following scale to determine rank:

U	S	A	E
0 to 28	29 to 50	51 to 76	77 to 96

Overall Performance Review Score _____.

ALL ITEMS IN THE FOLLOWING SECTION MUST BE COMPLETED:

A. Interviewer's comments on overall review _____
_____
_____

B. Additional suggestions for overall work improvement and goals for next evaluation _____
_____
_____

C. Self-objectives _____
_____
_____
_____

_____   _____
Date   Employee's signature

_____   _____
Date   Interviewer's signature

_____   _____
Date   Director of Nursing

INTENSIVE AND CORONARY CARE LICENSED PRACTICAL NURSE: JOB DESCRIPTION

Position Requirements:	Graduate from an accredited school for Licensed Practical Nurses with current licensure in the State of Alabama.
Professional Requirements:	Pursues programs of continuing education, participates in educational conferences, and updates and maintains knowledge and skills related to areas of practice.
Position Accountable for:	All nursing care behaviors described in the Intensive and Coronary Care Licensed Practical Nurse job description.
Position Accountable to:	Registered Nurse in charge of unit, Supervisor, Director of Nursing, patient and family.
Position Summary:	Performs the functions of a Licensed Practical Nurse in assessing, planning, implementing, and evaluating all assigned patient care in collaboration with the Registered Nurse in the unit. Is accountable for all patient care she gives during a shift. Is responsible for adhering to all Standards of Nursing Practice, for managing supplies and equipment with the direction of the Registered Nurse in charge of the unit, and for promoting teamwork with physicians and personnel of other departments.

I. *Assessment*
1. Assesses nursing care given by self; identifies problems and/or need for improvement and communicates this information to the RN in charge.
2. Assesses the health status of patients included in her assignment as outlined in Nursing Standards.
    2.1 Completes those portions of the patient assessment as directed by the Registered Nurse and Supervisor.
    2.2 Collects data from the patient, family and significant others, health care providers, individuals, and/or agencies in the community.
    2.3 Collects data by: interview, observation, inspection, auscultation, palpation, and reports and records.
    2.4 Organizes assessment data so that they are accurate, complete, accessible, and so that they remain confidential.
    2.5 Communicates assessment data in an orderly fashion by recording, updating, and communicating to the Registered Nurse and by revising as appropriate.

   2.6 Interprets heart patterns on monitor and assesses changes in pattern, verbalizes this to the Registered Nurse.

II. *Planning*
   1. Reviews and revises policies and procedures when requested.
   2. Plans and develops self-objectives with Supervisor, in conjunction with performance evaluation.
   3. Suggests ways to solve problems and to make improvements in the unit.
   4. In collaboration with the Registered Nurse, contributes to the formulation of assigned patient care plans, as outlined in the nursing standards.
      4.1 Identifies patient problems.
      4.2 Formulates desired outcomes.
      4.3 Communicates the above to the Registered Nurse.
      4.4 Participates with Registered Nurse in incorporating home health care into desired outcomes.

III. *Implementation*
   1. Implements activities necessary to meeting self-objectives.
   2. Cooperates with the Registered Nurse in implementing planned changes and activities to improve nursing care in the unit.
   3. Promotes harmonious relationships and favorable attitudes among the health care team.
   4. Supports and adheres to administrative and nursing service policies and procedures.
   5. Assists with orientation of new employees.
   6. Attends required inservice education programs.
   7. Participates with Registered Nurse in the unit in the implementation of assigned patients care plans.
   8. Documents nursing actions implemented, and effectiveness of implementation, in the nurses' notes in a continuous manner.
   9. In the event the Registered Nurse is responding to Code "9" (cardiac arrest) within the hospital, assists authorized personnel during her absence from unit.
   10. Is knowledgeable of location, care, and operation of Intensive Care Unit equipment. This includes but is not limited to: monitors, defibrillation equipment, crash carts and contents, trays (trachea, CVP), pacemaker, and ventilator.
   11. Manages self and assists with management of assigned patients during emergencies.
   12. Maintains clean, organized unit and restocks supplies as necessary.
   13. Provides a calm, reassuring atmosphere and communicates effectively with each patient's family to reduce stress.
   14. Conforms to hospital dress code.
   15. Is rarely sick or absent from work due to health.
   16. Is prompt and attends report.

IV. *Evaluation*

1. Evaluates the nursing care she gives.
2. Evaluates self-objectives and determines need for new objectives.
3. Evaluates the effectiveness of problem-solving techniques and activities implemented to improve nursing care in the unit.
4. Evaluates LPN orientation policies and procedures and recommends revisions.
5. Participates in the evaluation of inservice education programs.
6. Participates with the Registered Nurse in the evaluation and revision of assigned patients' care plans.

INTENSIVE AND CORONARY CARE LICENSED PRACTICAL NURSE: PERFORMANCE EVALUATION

Name _____ Employment Date _____

Rating Period _____ To _____

Department _____ Job Title _____

Instructions: Using the following rating scale, indicate the quality of performance by placing the appropriate letter on the line to the left of the item.

U*– Unsatisfactory (does not meet job requirements)
S – Satisfactory (meets job requirements)
A – Above average (exceeds job requirements)
E* – Exceptional performance

I. *Assessment:*

_____ 1. Assesses nursing care given by self; identifies problems and/or need for improvement and communicates this information to the RN in charge.

_____

_____

_____ 2. Assesses the health status of patients included in her assignment as outlined in Nursing Standards.
    2.1 Completes those portions of the patient assessment as directed by the Registered Nurse and Supervisor.

_____

_____

    2.2 Collects data from the patient, family and significant others, health care providers, individuals, and/or agencies in the community.

_____

_____

    2.3 Collects data by: interview, observation, inspection, auscultation, palpation, and reports and records.

_____

_____

_____

*The evaluator is expected to comment on all items rated "U" or "E."

144

2.4 Organizes assessment data so that they are accurate, complete, and accessible, and so that they remain confidential.

_____

_____

2.5 Communicates assessment data in an orderly fashion by recording, updating, and communicating to the Registered Nurse and revising as appropriate.

_____

_____

2.6 Interprets heart patterns on monitor and assesses changes in pattern, verbalizes this to the Registered Nurse.

_____

_____

II. _Planning:_

_____ 1. Reviews and revises policies and procedures when requested.

_____

_____

_____ 2. Plans and develops self-objectives with Supervisor in conjunction with performance evaluation.

_____

_____

_____ 3. Suggests ways to solve problems and to make improvements in the unit.

_____

_____

_____ 4. In collaboration with the Registered Nurse, contributes to the formulation of assigned patient care plans, as outlined in the Nursing Standards:
4.1 Identifies patient problems.

_____

_____

4.2 Formulates desired outcomes.

_____

_____

4.3 Communicates the above to the Registered Nurse.

_____

_____

4.4 Participates with Registered Nurse in incorporating home health care into desired outcomes.

_____

_____

III. *Implementation:*

_____ 1. Implements activities necessary to meeting self-objectives.

_____

_____

_____ 2. Cooperates with the Registered Nurse in implementing planned changes and activities to improve nursing care in the unit.

_____

_____

_____ 3. Promotes harmonious relationships and favorable attitudes among the health care team.

_____

_____

_____ 4. Supports and adheres to administrative and nursing service policies and procedures.

_____

_____

_____ 5. Assists with orientation of new employees.

_____

_____

_____ 6. Attends required inservice education programs.

_____

_____

_____ 7. Participates with Registered Nurse in the unit in the implementation of assigned patients' care plans.

_____

_____

_____ 8. Documents nursing actions implemented and effectiveness of implementation in the nurses' notes in a continuous manner.

_____

_____

_____ 9. In the event the Registered Nurse is responding to Code "9" (cardiac arrest) within the hospital, assists authorized personnel during her absence from the unit.

_____

_____

_____ 10. Is knowledgeable of location, care, and operation of Intensive Care Unit equipment. This includes but is not limited to: monitors, defibrillation equipment, crash carts and contents, trays (trachea, CVP), pacemaker, and ventilator.

_____

_____

_____ 11. Manages self and assists with management of assigned patients during emergencies.

_____

_____

_____ 12. Maintains clean, organized unit and restocks supplies as necessary.

_____

_____

_____ 13. Provides a calm, reassuring atmosphere and communicates effectively with each patient's family to reduce stress.

_____

_____

_____ 14. Conforms to hospital dress code.

_____

_____

_____ 15. Is rarely sick or absent from work due to health.

_____

_____

_____ 16. Is prompt and attends report.

_____

_____

IV. _Evaluation:_

_____ 1. Evaluates the nursing care she gives.

_____

_____

_____ 2. Evaluates self-objectives and determines need for new objectives.

_____

_____

_____ 3. Evaluates the effectiveness of problem-solving techniques and activities implemented to improve nursing care in the unit.

_____

_____

_____ 4. Evaluates LPN orientation policies and procedures and recommends revisions.

_____

_____

_____ 5. Participates in the evaluation of inservice education programs.

_____

_____

_____ 6. Participates with the Registered Nurse in the evaluation and revision of assigned patients' care plans.

_____

_____

INTENSIVE AND CORONARY CARE LICENSED PRACTICAL NURSE: SCORING PROCEDURE

Instructions: Total the number of each item and multiply times the appropriate number. Add these totals to make the score.

U _____ × 0 = _____

S _____ × 1 = _____

A _____ × 2 = _____

E _____ × 3 = _____   _____ Total Score

Compare total score to the following scale to determine rank:

U	S	A	E
0 to 24	25 to 44	45 to 66	67 to 84

Overall Performance Review Score _____.

ALL ITEMS IN THE FOLLOWING SECTION MUST BE COMPLETED:

A. Interviewer's comments on overall review _____
_____
_____

B. Additional suggestions for overall work improvement and goals for next evaluation _____
_____
_____

C. Self-objectives _____
_____
_____
_____

_____   _____
Date   Employee's signature

_____   _____
Date   Interviewer's signature

_____   _____
Date   Director of Nursing

9
Surgical Nursing Practice

STANDARDS OF SURGICAL NURSING PRACTICE

STANDARD I

Assessment is the identification and gathering of data concerning the health status of the patient. This process is complete, continuous, and systematic as evidenced by:

1. *A complete patient history and physical pertinent to the surgical procedure:*
   a. *Patient interview:*
      Chief complaint
      History of present illness
      Allergies
      Medications
      Past medical/surgical history
      Family history
      Preferred name (nickname)
      Nutritional status
      Prosthesis
      Identification of patient
      Activities of daily living
      Cultural and socioeconomic conditions
      Personal habits
      Food and fluid preferences
      Appetite changes/weight changes
      Pattern of communication
   b. *Psychological assessment:*
      Emotional status
      Patterns of coping
      Concerns during or dealing with surgical procedure
      Perception of surgical procedure
      Understanding of surgical procedure
      Understanding of reason for surgical procedure
      Desired outcome from surgical procedure
      Body image
      Knowledge of expected behaviors following surgical procedure
   c. *Physical assessment:*
      Personal hygiene
      Complete and accurate skin prep for surgical procedure
      Systems review:
      1. *Respiratory:*
         Respiratory-rate and quality
         Dyspnea
         Orthopnea
         Cough
         Sputum
         Breath sounds

2. *Cardiovascular:*
   Heart rate and quality
   Arrhythmias
   Varicosities
   Peripheral pulses
   Edema

3. *Skin:*
   Petechiae
   Color
   Moisture level
   Temperature
   Nail beds
   Turgor

4. *Chest:*
   Breast
   Discharge
   Lumps
   Bleeding
   Nipple retraction

5. *Gastrointestinal:*
   Nausea/vomiting
   Recent weight loss or gain
   Distention
   Tarry stools
   Hard abdomen
   Diarrhea
   Constipation
   Bowel sounds:
   a. Hypoactive
   b. Hyperactive
   c. Absent
   Last bowel movement

6. *Musculoskeletal:*
   Back pain
   Neck pain
   Extremity pain
   Joint swelling
   Fractures
   Range of motion

7. *Mental/neurological:*
   Syncope
   Seizure
   Restlessness
   Dizziness
   Headache
   Paralysis
   Lethargic
   Semicomatose

Comatose

Confused

8. *Genitourinary*

Dysuria

Frequency

Burning

Nocturia

Hematuria

Incontinence

Retention

Male:

a. Prostate problems

Female:

a. LMP

b. Vaginal discharge

c. Unusual vaginal bleeding

2. *The collection of data from available sources:*

Patient, family, significant others

Health care providers

3. *The collection of data by scientific methodology:*

Interview

Observation

Inspection

Auscultation

Palpation

4. *The collection of data by interpretation/assessment of reports and records:*

Identification of patient

Consent form

Preanesthesia evaluation

History and physical

Confirmation of surgical site

Vital signs (time taken)

Preoperative medication (time given)

Urinalysis

Hematology studies

EKG

Doctor's order

Radiological studies

Last oral intake

Time of last voiding

Any other studies required

5. *The organization of data in a systematic arrangement:*

The arrangement provides:

a. Accurate collection

b. Complete collection

c. Accessibility

d. Confidentiality

6. *The communication of data in an orderly fashion:*
   Data are recorded preoperatively, intraoperatively, and postoperatively.
   Data are updated preoperatively, intraoperatively, and postoperatively.
   Data are revised and recorded as appropriate.
   Data are communicated verbally among health team.

STANDARD II

Nursing care planning consists of determining patient problems and desired outcomes. Planning involves preparing the patient for the surgical procedure—both pre and postoperatively. Planning involves maintaining bio-psycho-social status, preoperatively, intraoperatively, and postoperatively. This is evidenced by:

1. *The identification of present/potential patient problems, from the patient assessment:*
   Data are grouped into meaningful arrangement, based upon scientific knowledge.
   Patient's health status is determined.
   Patient's health status is compared to the norms.
   Present and potential problems are identified.
   Problems are given priority according to impact upon the patient's health status.
2. *The formulation of desired outcomes:*
   Patient (family, significant other) and nurse mutually agree upon the patient's present/potential health problems.
   Patient and nurse mutually agree upon desired outcomes.
   Desired outcomes are congruent with the patient problems and established norms.
   Desired outcomes are specific.
   Desired outcomes are measurable within a certain time frame.
   Desired outcomes are consistent with other health providers' expectations.
   Desired outcomes are established to restore patient's optimal functioning capabilities.
3. *The incorporation of postoperative care into desired outcomes. This involves preoperative teaching:*
   Explanation of surgical procedure.
   Medication—preoperative medications, pain medication, and postoperative medications.
   Diet: (i.e., NPO) plan for progression following the procedure.
   Exercise/activity: cough, turn and deep-breathing technique, ambulation, and other expected behaviors or limitations.
   Explanation of any extraneous equipment necessary following the procedure (i.e., IV, nasogastric tube, Foley catheter, hemovac drain).
   Self-care techniques and materials.
   Available support systems, health information and resources that will enable the patient to understand and accept necessary modifications in body image and/or life-style.

STANDARD III

The plan of care is implemented in order to achieve the desired outcome. This is evidenced by:

1. *The formulation of nursing prescriptions that delineate actions to be taken:*
   Prescribed actions:
   Are specific to identified patient problems and desired outcomes.
   Are based on current scientific knowledge.
   Incorporate principles of preoperative patient teaching.
   Incorporate principles of psychosocial interactions.
   Include human, material, and support systems.
   Include keeping patient/family/significant other knowledgeable of health status and total health care plan.
2. *The implementation of actions delineated in the nursing prescriptions:*
   Actions implemented:
   Actively involve the patient and family.
   Are consistent with the nursing prescriptions.
   Are based upon current scientific knowledge.
   Are flexible and individualized for each patient.
   Provide patient privacy and dignity.
3. *The implementation of all nursing actions reflect:*
   Environmental factors that influence the patient's health (i.e., anesthetics, equipment, etc.).
   Principles of infection control (i.e., traffic control, control of contaminants, and sterile and aseptic techniques).
   Principles of safety (i.e., transfer of patient, positioning of patient, electrical safety, etc.).

Standard IV

Outcomes of Nursing Actions are evaluated for further assessment and planning. This is evidenced by:

1. *Evaluating the achievement of desired outcomes:*
   Data are collected concerning the patient's health status.
   Data are compared to the specific desired outcomes.
   The patient and nurse evaluate the achievement of desired outcomes.
2. *Reassessment of the nursing care plan:*
   Outcome of nursing actions direct the reassessment of identified patient problems.
   Outcome of nursing actions direct assessment of desired outcomes (assess the desired outcome to determine if appropriate, realistic, and in correct priority).
   Outcome of nursing actions direct reassessment of nursing prescriptions (assess the nursing prescriptions to determine if appropriate, realistic, and stated accurately).
   Nursing actions are assessed for effectiveness in achieving desired outcomes.

3. *Further planning as directed by the reassessment:*

Reassessment determines new patient present/potential problems.

New patient problems direct the formulation and revision of desired outcomes.

Revised desired outcomes direct the revising of nursing prescriptions.

Revised prescriptions direct new actions to be implemented toward desired outcomes.

Desired outcomes are continually evaluated for achievement.

The plan of care is continually evaluated and revised according to changes in the patient's health status.

SURGICAL SUPERVISOR: JOB DESCRIPTION

Position Requirements:	Graduate from an accredited school of nursing with current licensure as a registered nurse in the State of Alabama. Five years recent clinical experience in Operating Room/Recovery Room, including at least 1 year supervisory experience.
Professional Requirements:	Pursues programs of continuing education consistent with requirements of the Alabama Nurses' Association. Participates in educational conferences and updates and maintains professional knowledge and skills related to the management of areas of responsibility.
Position Accountable for:	All nursing care behaviors described in the Surgical Supervisor job description.
Position Accountable to:	Director of Nursing Service, the patient, and family.
Position Summary:	Performs the primary functions of a professional nurse leader in assessing, planning, implementing, directing, and evaluating the care of all patients in Operating Room/Recovery Room on a 24-hour basis. Is responsible for meeting the Joint Commission Standards of patient care as well as the established Surgical Standards of Nursing Practice, for managing all assigned personnel, supplies, and equipment in the Operating Room/Recovery Room, and for promoting teamwork with physicians and personnel of other departments.

I. *Assessment*

1. Assesses the number and level of personnel needed to provide quality patient care and adjusts staffing and assignments appropriately.
2. Assesses surgical department functions and activities as related to other hospital departments.
3. Assesses the delivery of nursing care and identifies problems and any need for improvement.
4. Ensures the collection and documentation of a patient assessment prior to the surgical procedure.
5. Ensures that the health status of all patients is assessed as outlined in the Standards of Surgical Nursing Practice and under hospital policy prior to the surgical procedures.

Ensures that:

5.1 A complete history and physical pertinent to the surgical procedure is taken. This includes but is not limited to:
   a. Site preparation for surgical procedure
   b. Patterns of communication
   c. Preferred nickname
   d. Nutritional status
   e. Emotional status
   f. Patterns of coping
   g. Patient's concerns during or dealing with surgical procedure
   h. Patient's understanding of surgical procedure
   i. Patient's desired outcomes from surgical procedure
   j. Patient's perception of body image
   k. Patient's understanding of behaviors expected following surgical procedure

5.2 Data are collected from patient, family and significant others, and health care providers.

5.3 Data are collected by interview, observation, inspection, auscultation, and palpation.

5.4 Reports and records are assessed and interpreted, and pertinent information is verbalized among health team members: (a) accurate identification of patient, (b) complete consent form, (c) vital signs (and time), (d) preanesthesia evaluation, (e) confirmation of surgical site, (f) preoperative medication (and time), (g) CBC, U/A, EKG and CXR, and other lab and x-ray reports, (h) last oral intake, (i) time of last voiding, and (j) other pertinent reports.

5.5 Ensures that assessment data are organized so that they are accurate, complete, and accessible, and so that they remain confidential.

5.6 Ensures that assessment data are communicated in an orderly fashion among the health team preoperatively, intraoperatively, and postoperatively and are recorded and revised appropriately.

II. *Planning*

1. Serves on hospital committees as requested.

2. Develops, reviews, and revises all policies and procedures for Operating Room/Recovery Room with approval from Director of Nursing.

3. Plans and develops self-objectives.

4. Plans ways to solve problems and to make improvements in the delivery of patient care in collaboration with Director of Nursing.

5. Ensures that all patients have a written nursing care plan. Establishes individual patient's care plans as well as directs and supervises others in the formulation of patient care plans.

   Ensures that:

   5.1 The patient's present/potential problems are identified from the patient assessment.
      a. Patient's health status is determined,
      b. Health status is compared to the norms,

     c. Problems are given priority according to impact upon the patient's health status.

  5.2 Desired outcomes are formulated specific to the patient problems and established norms.

  5.3 Ensures that desired outcomes are mutually agreed upon by the patient and nurse and are: (a) specific, (b) measureable within a certain time frame, and (c) consistent with other health providers' expectations.

6. Ensures the incorporation of postoperative care into expected outcomes, by preoperative teaching (including but not limited to):

  6.1 Explanation of surgical procedure.

  6.2 Medication—preoperative medications, pain medication, and postoperative medications.

  6.3 Diet (i.e., NPO) plan for progression following the procedure.

  6.4 Exercise/activity: cough, turn and deep-breathing techniques, ambulation, and other expected behaviors or limitations.

  6.5 Explanation of any extraneous equipment necessary following the procedure (i.e., IV, nasogastric tube, Foley catheter, hemovac drain).

  6.6 Self-care techniques and materials.

  6.7 Available support systems health information and resources that will enable the patient to understand and accept necessary modifications in body image and/or life-style.

III. *Implementation*

1. Implements activities necessary to meeting self-objectives.

2. Promotes the achievement of Operating/Recovery Room objectives.

3. Directs, supervises, and participates in implementing planned changes and activities to improve the department in collaboration with Director of Nursing and Medical Director.

4. Ensures that Standards of Surgical Nursing Practice are implemented, and assists in monitoring of standards as necessary.

5. Holds self and staff accountable for the delivery of quality nursing care.

6. Acts rapidly and effectively, follows hospital policies and procedures, and utilizes principles of management in any emergency situation.

7. Promotes harmonious relationships and favorable attitudes among the health care team.

8. Interprets, supports, and recommends administrative and nursing service policies and procedures for employees. Applies knowledge and skills of management.

9. Directs and assists with orientation of new employees.

10. Keeps the Director of Nursing Service informed on reportable situations and nursing unit needs.

11. Attends required inservice education programs.

12. Ensures that nursing prescriptions are formulated as outlined in the nursing standards that delineate actions to be taken. Ensures that prescribed actions:

12.1 Are specific to the patient's problems and the desired outcomes.

12.2 Are based on scientific knowledge.

12.3 Incorporate principles of preoperative patient teaching.

12.4 Incorporate principles of psychosocial interactions.

12.5 Include human, material, and community resources.

12.6 Include keeping patient knowledgeable of health status and total health care plan.

13. Ensures that the actions delineated in the nursing prescriptions are implemented. Actions implemented:

13.1 Actively involve the patient and family.

13.2 Are based on current scientific knowledge.

13.3 Are flexible and individualized for each patient.

13.4 Provide patient privacy and dignity.

13.5 Incorporate principles of safety.

13.6 Incorporate principles of infection control.

13.7 Reflect environmental factors affecting patient's health.

14. Serves as consultant in technical and professional matters for personnel.

15. Participates and contributes to a unified Quality Assurance Program.

16. Participates in the provision of inservice education programs pertinent to surgical department.

17. Demonstrates knowledge of and skill in exercising all Operating Room/Recovery Room procedures.

18. Demonstrates knowledge of location, care, and use of all equipment/supplies pertaining to Operating Room/Recovery Room.

19. Demonstrates knowledge of sterile/aseptic technique and recognizes and corrects any breaks in this technique.

20. Is always available and accessible when on duty or on call.

21. Conforms to hospital dress code.

22. Is rarely sick or absent from work due to health.

23. Is prompt.

IV. *Evaluation*

1. Continually evaluates Standards of Surgical Nursing Practice by reviewing nursing care plans, assessing patients, reviewing charts, interviewing, observing, participating in Quality Assurance activities, by employing other means of evaluation. Revises standards as appropriate in collaboration with Director of Nursing.

2. Evaluates policies and procedures and revises as necessary.

3. Evaluates self-objectives and determines need for revision and new objectives.

4. Evaluates the effectiveness of problem-solving techniques and activities implemented to improve the department.

5. Evaluates the performance of Operating Room/Recovery Room nursing personnel.

6. Evaluates the achievement of Surgical Nursing objectives.

7. Evaluates emergencies and any hospital disaster and recommends revisions in policies and procedures and/or need for improvement in employee performance.

8. Evaluates orientation policies and procedures and recommends revisions as necessary.

9. Evaluates inservice education programs.

10. Ensures that desired outcomes are evaluated for achievement or lack of achievement.
    10.1 Data are collected concerning the patient's health status.
    10.2 Data are compared to the specific desired outcomes.
    10.3 The patient and nurse evaluate the achievement of desired outcomes.

11. Ensures that the nursing care plans are reassessed and revised according to the evaluation of achievement or lack of achievement of desired outcomes.

    From evaluation:
    11.1 Reassesses the patient problems.
    11.2 Reassesses desired outcomes to determine if appropriate, realistic, and in correct priority.
    11.3 Reassesses nursing prescriptions to determine if appropriate, realistic, and stated accurately.
    11.4 Reassesses nursing actions for effectiveness in achieving desired outcomes.

    From reassessment:
    11.5 New patient present/potential problems are determined.
    11.6 From new patient problems desired outcomes are formulated and revised.
    11.7 Nursing prescriptions are revised.
    11.8 New actions are implemented in order to carry out revised prescriptions.
    11.9 Desired outcomes are continually evaluated for achievement or lack of achievement.
    11.10 The nursing care plan is continually evaluated and revised according to changes in the patient's health status.

SURGICAL SUPERVISOR: PERFORMANCE EVALUATION

Name _____ Employment Date _____

Rating Period _____ To _____

Department _____ Job Title _____

Instructions: Using the following rating scale, indicate the quality of performance by placing the appropriate letter on the line to the left of the item.

U* – Unsatisfactory (does not meet job requirements)
S – Satisfactory (meets job requirements)
A – Above average (exceeds job requirements)
E* – Exceptional performance

I. *Assessment:*

_____ 1. Assesses the number and level of personnel needed to provide quality patient care and adjusts staffing and assignments appropriately.

_____
_____

_____ 2. Assesses surgical department functions and activities as related to other hospital departments.

_____
_____

_____ 3. Assesses the delivery of nursing care and identifies problems and any need for improvement.

_____
_____

_____ 4. Ensures the collection and documentation of a patient assessment prior to the surgical procedure.

_____
_____

_____ 5. Ensures that the health status of all patients is assessed as outlined in the Standards of Surgical Nursing Practice and under hospital policy prior to the surgical procedures.
Ensures that:
5.1 A complete history and physical pertinent to the surgical procedure is taken. This includes but is not limited to:

---

*The evaluator is expected to comment on all items rated "U" or "E."

a. Site preparation for surgical procedure
b. Patterns of communication
c. Preferred nickname
d. Nutritional status
e. Emotional status
f. Patterns of coping
g. Patient's concerns during or dealing with surgical procedure
h. Patient's understanding of surgical procedure
i. Patient's desired outcomes from surgical procedure
j. Patient's perception of body image
k. Patient's understanding of behaviors expected following surgical procedure

5.2 Data are collected from patient, family and significant others, and health care providers.

5.3 Data are collected by interview, observation, inspection, auscultation, and palpation.

5.4 Reports and records are assessed and interpreted, and pertinent information is verbalized among health team members:
a. Accurate identification of patient
b. Complete consent form
c. Vital signs (and time)
d. Preanesthesia evaluation
e. Confirmation of surgical site
f. Preoperative medication (and time)
g. CBC, U/A, EKG and CXR, and other lab and x-ray reports
h. Last oral intake
i. Time of last voiding
j. Other pertinent reports

5.5 Ensures that assessment data are organized so that they are accurate, complete, accessible, and so that they remain confidential.

5.6 Ensures that assessment data are communicated in an orderly fashion among the health team preoperatively, intraoperatively, and postoperatively and is recorded and revised appropriately.

_____

_____

II. *Planning:*

_____ 1. Serves on hospital committees as requested.

_____

_____

_____ 2. Develops, reviews, and revises all policies and procedures for Operating Room/Recovery Room with approval from Director of Nursing.

_____

_____

_____ 3. Plans and develops self-objectives.

_____

_____

_____ 4. Plans ways to solve problems and to make improvements in the delivery of patient care in collaboration with Director of Nursing.

_____

_____

_____ 5. Ensures that all patients have a written nursing care plan. Establishes individual patient's care plans as well as directs and supervises others in the formulation of patient care plans. Ensures that:

5.1 The patient's present/potential problems are identified from the patient assessment:
   a. Patient's health status is determined,
   b. Health status is compared to the norms,
   c. Problems are given priority according to impact upon the patient's health status.

_____

_____

5.2 Desired outcomes are formulated specific to the patient problems and established norms.

_____

_____

5.3 Ensures that desired outcomes are mutually agreed upon by the patient and nurse and are:

a. Specific
b. Measurable within a certain time frame
c. Consistent with other health providers' expectations

_____

_____

_____ 6. Ensures the incorporation of postoperative care into expected outcomes by preoperative teaching, including but not limited to:
6.1 Explanation of surgical procedure.

_____

6.2 Medication—preoperative medications, pain medication, and postoperative medications.

_____

6.3 Diet (i.e., NPO) plan for progression following the procedure.

_____

6.4 Exercise/activity: cough, turn and deep-breathing techniques, ambulation, and other expected behaviors or limitations.

_____

6.5 Explanation of any extraneous equipment necessary following the procedure (i.e., IV, nasogastric tube, Foley catheter, hemovac drain).

_____

6.6 Self-care techniques and materials.

_____

6.7 Available support systems health information and resources that will enable the patient to understand and accept necessary modifications in body image and/or life-style.

_____

_____

III. *Implementation:*

_____ 1. Implements activities necessary to meeting self-objectives.

_____

_____

_____ 2. Promotes the achievement of Operating/Recovery Room objectives.

_____

_____

_____ 3. Directs, supervises, and participates in implementing planned changes and activities to improve the department in collaboration with Director of Nursing and Medical Director.

_____

_____

_____ 4. Ensures that Standards of Surgical Nursing Practice are implemented and assists in monitoring of standards as necessary.

_____

_____

_____ 5. Holds self and staff accountable for the delivery of quality nursing care.

_____

_____

_____ 6. Acts rapidly and effectively, follows hospital policies and procedures, and utilizes principles of management in any emergency situation.

_____

_____

_____ 7. Promotes harmonious relationships and favorable attitudes among the health care team.

_____

_____

_____ 8. Interprets, supports, and recommends administrative and nursing service policies and procedures for employees. Applies knowledge and skills of management.

_____

_____

_____ 9. Directs and assists with orientation of new employees.

_____

_____

_____ 10. Keeps the Director of Nursing Service informed on reportable situations and nursing unit needs.

_____

_____

_____ 11. Attends required inservice education programs.

_____

_____

_____ 12. Ensures that nursing prescriptions are formulated as outlined in the nursing standards that delineate actions to be taken. Ensures that prescribed actions:
   12.1 Are specific to the patient's problems and the desired outcomes.

   _____

   _____

   12.2 Are based on scientific knowledge.

   _____

   12.3 Incorporate principles of preoperative patient teaching.

   _____

   12.4 Incorporate principles of psychosocial interactions.

   _____

   12.5 Include human, material, and community resources.

   _____

   12.6 Include keeping patient knowledgeable of health status and total health care plan.

   _____

   _____

_____ 13. Ensures that the actions delineated in the nursing prescriptions are implemented. Actions implemented:
   13.1 Actively involve the patient and family.

   _____

   13.2 Are based on current scientific knowledge.

   _____

   13.3 Are flexible and individualized for each patient.

   _____

   _____

13.4 Provide patient privacy and dignity.

_____

_____

13.5 Incorporate principles of safety.

_____

_____

13.6 Incorporate principles of infection control.

_____

_____

13.7 Reflect environmental factors affecting patient's health.

_____

_____

_____ 14. Serves as consultant in technical and professional matters for personnel.

_____

_____

_____ 15. Participates and contributes to a unified Quality Assurance Program.

_____

_____

_____ 16. Participates in the provision of inservice education programs pertinent to surgical department.

_____

_____

_____ 17. Demonstrates knowledge of and skill in exercising all Operating Room/Recovery Room procedures.

_____

_____

_____ 18. Demonstrates knowledge of location, care, and use of all equipment and supplies pertaining to Operating Room/Recovery Room.

_____

_____

_____ 19. Demonstrates knowledge of sterile/aseptic technique and recognizes and corrects any breaks in this technique.

_____

_____

_____ 20. Is always available and accessible when on duty or on call.

_____ 21. Conforms to hospital dress code.

_____ 22. Is rarely sick or absent from work due to health.

_____ 23. Is prompt.

IV. *Evaluation:*

_____ 1. Continually evaluates Standards of Surgical Nursing Practice by reviewing nursing care plans, assessing patients, reviewing charts, interviewing, observing, participating in Quality Assurance activities, and by employing other means of evaluation. Revises standards as appropriate in collaboration with Director of Nursing.

_____ 2. Evaluates policies and procedures and revises as necessary.

_____ 3. Evaluates self-objectives and determines need for revision and new objectives.

_____ 4. Evaluates the effectiveness of problem-solving techniques and activities implemented to improve the department.

_____ 5. Evaluates the performance of Operating Room/Recovery Room nursing personnel.

_____ 6. Evaluates the achievement of Surgical Nursing objectives.

_____

_____

_____ 7. Evaluates emergencies and any hospital disaster and recommends revisions in policies and procedures and/or need for improvement in employee performance.

_____

_____

_____ 8. Evaluates orientation policies and procedures and recommends revisions as necessary.

_____

_____

_____ 9. Evaluates inservice education programs.

_____

_____

_____ 10. Ensures that desired outcomes are evaluated for achievement or lack of achievement:
10.1 Data are collected concerning the patient's health status.

_____

10.2 Data are compared to the specific desired outcomes.

_____

10.3 The patient and nurse evaluate the achievement of desired outcomes.

_____

_____ 11. Ensures that the nursing care plans are reassessed and revised according to the evaluation of achievement or lack of achievement of desired outcomes.
From evaluation:
11.1   Reassesses the patient problems.

_____

11.2   Reassesses desired outcomes to determine if appropriate, realistic, and in correct priority.

_____

_____

11.3　Reassesses nursing prescriptions to determine if appropriate, realistic, and stated accurately.

_____

11.4　Reassesses nursing actions for effectiveness in achieving desired outcomes.

_____

From reassessment:

11.5　New patient present/potential problems are determined.

_____

11.6　From new patient problems desired outcomes are formulated and revised.

_____

11.7　Nursing prescriptions are revised.

_____

11.8　New actions are implemented in order to carry out revised prescriptions.

_____

11.9　Desired outcomes are continually evaluated for achievement or lack of achievement.

_____

11.10　The nursing care plan is continually evaluated and revised according to changes in the patient's health status.

_____

SURGICAL SUPERVISOR: SCORING PROCEDURE

Instructions: Total the number of each item and multiply times the appropriate number. Add these totals to make the score.

U _____×0=_____

S _____×1=_____

A _____×2=_____

E _____×3=_____   _____ Total Score

Compare total score to the following scale to determine rank:

U	S	A	E
0 to 40	41 to 71	72 to 107	108 to 135

Overall Performance Review Score _____

ALL ITEMS IN THE FOLLOWING SECTION MUST BE COMPLETED:

A. Interviewer's comments on overall review _____

_____

_____

B. Additional suggestions for overall work improvement and goals for next evaluation _____

_____

_____

C. Self-objectives _____

_____

_____

_____

_____   _____

Date   Employee's signature

_____   _____

Date   Interviewer's signature

_____   _____

Date   Director of Nursing

SURGICAL REGISTERED NURSE: JOB DESCRIPTION

Position Requirements: Graduate from an accredited school of nursing with current licensure as a registered nurse in the State of Alabama. Specific orientation for Operating Room/Recovery Room nursing.

Professional Requirements: Pursues programs of continuing education consistent with requirements of the Alabama Nurses' Association. Participates in educational conferences and updates and maintains professional knowledge and skills related to areas of responsibility.

Position Accountable for: All nursing care behaviors described in the Surgical Registered Nurse (Operating Room/Recovery Room) job description.

Position Accountable to: Surgical Supervisor, Director of Nursing, the patient, and family.

Position Summary: Performs the primary functions of a Registered Nurse in assessing, planning, implementing, and evaluating the care of all assigned patients in Operating Room/Recovery Room during her shift. Is responsible for meeting the established Surgical Standards of Nursing Practice, for managing all assigned personnel, supplies, and equipment in the Operating Room/Recovery Room, and for promoting teamwork with physicians and personnel of other departments.

I. *Assessment*
   1. Assesses the number and level of personnel needed to provide quality patient care in the department and collaborates with the Supervisor in adjusting staffing and assignments.
   2. Participates in the assessment of functions and activities in Operating Room/Recovery Room as they relate to other departments.
   3. Assesses the delivery of nursing care in the department and identifies problems and any need for improvements.
   4. Assesses the health status of all patients, as outlined in the Standards of Surgical Nursing Practice and under hospital policy, prior to the surgical procedure.
      4.1 Completes a patient history and physical pertinent to the surgical procedure but is not limited to:
         a. Site preparation for surgical procedure
         b. Patterns of communication

174

  c. Preferred nickname

  d. Nutritional status

  e. Emotional status

  f. Patterns of coping

  g. Patient's concerns during or dealing with surgical procedure

  h. Patient's understanding of surgical procedure

  i. Patient's expected outcomes from surgical procedure

  j. Patient's perception of body image

  k. Patient's understanding of behaviors expected following surgical procedure

 4.2 Collects data from patient, family and significant others, and health care providers.

 4.3 Collects data by interview, observation, inspection, auscultation, and palpation.

 4.4 Assesses and interprets reports and records, verbalizes pertinent information among health team members: (a) accurate identification of patient, (b) complete consent form, (c) preanethesia evaluation, (d) confirmation of surgical site, (e) vital signs (and time), (f) preoperative medications (and time), (g) CBC, U/A, EKG and CXR, and other lab or x-ray reports, (h) last oral intake, (i) time of last voiding, and (j) other pertinent reports.

 4.5 Organizes assessment data so that they are accurate, complete, and accessible, and so that they remain confidential.

 4.6 Communicates assessment data in an orderly fashion among the health team preoperatively, intraoperatively, and postoperatively and records and revises appropriately.

II. *Planning*

 1. Serves on hospital committees as requested.

 2. Participates in developing, reviewing, and revising policies and procedures as directed by Supervisor.

 3. Plans and develops self-objectives.

 4. Plans ways to solve problems and to make improvements in the department in collaboration with the Supervisor.

 5. Completes a written care plan for assigned patients. Plans the care for individual patients as well as directs and supervises others in the planning of patient's care.

  5.1 Identifies the patient's present/potential problems from the patient assessment.

   a. patient's health status is determined,

   b. health status is compared to the norms,

   c. problems are given priority according to impact upon the patient's health status.

  5.2 Formulates desired outcomes, specific to the patient problems and established norms.

  5.3 Ensures that desired outcomes are mutually agreed upon by the patient and nurse and are: (a) specific, (b) measureable within a certain time frame, and (c) consistent with other health providers' expectations.

6. Incorporates postoperative care into expected outcomes by preoperative teaching (including but not limited to):
   6.1 Explanation of surgical procedure.
   6.2 Medication—preoperative medications, pain medications, and post-operative medications.
   6.3 Diet (i.e., NPO) plan for progression following the procedure.
   6.4 Exercise/Activity: cough, turn and deep-breathing techniques, ambulation, and other expected behaviors or limitations.
   6.5 Explanation of any extraneous equipment necessary following the procedure (i.e., IV, nasogastric tube, Foley catheter, hemovac drain).
   6.6 Self-care techniques and materials.
   6.7 Available support systems, health information, and resources that will enable the patient to understand and accept necessary modifications in body image and/or life-style.

III. *Implementation*
   1. Implements activities necessary to meeting self-objectives.
   2. Participates in implementing planned changes, and activities to improve the department.
   3. Holds self and staff accountable for the delivery of quality nursing care.
   4. Promotes harmonious relationships and favorable attitudes among the health care team.
   5. Supports and adheres to nursing service and administrative policies and procedures.
   6. Assists with orientation of new employees.
   7. Acts rapidly and effectively, manages self, patients, and other employees during any emergency situation.
   8. Attends required inservice education programs.
   9. Formulates nursing prescriptions that delineate actions to be taken. Prescribed actions:
      9.1 Are specific to the patient's problems and desired outcomes.
      9.2 Are based on scientific knowledge.
      9.3 Are based on principles of psychosocial interactions.
      9.4 Are based on principles of preoperative patient teaching.
      9.5 Include human, material, and community resources.
      9.6 Include keeping patient knowledgeable of health status and total health care plan.
   10. Implements the actions delineated in the nursing prescriptions. Actions implemented:
      10.1 Actively involve the patient and family.
      10.2 Are based on current scientific knowledge.
      10.3 Are flexible and individualized for each patient.
      10.4 Provide patient privacy and dignity.
      10.5 Incorporate principles of safety.
      10.6 Incorporate principles of infection control.
      10.7 Reflect environmental factors affecting patient's health.

11. Demonstrates knowledge of and skill in exercising all Operating Room/Recovery Room procedures.
12. Demonstrates knowledge of location, care, and use of all equipment/supplies pertaining to Operating Room/Recovery Room.
13. Demonstrates knowledge of sterile/aseptic technique and recognizes and corrects any breaks in this technique.
14. Is always available and accessible when on duty or on call.
15. Conforms to hospital dress code.
16. Is rarely sick or absent from work due to health.
17. Is prompt.

IV. *Evaluation*
1. Evaluates Operating Room/Recovery Room policies and procedures and recommends the need for revision as assigned by Supervisor.
2. Evaluates self-objectives and determines need for revisions and new objectives.
3. Evaluates the effectiveness of problem-solving techniques and the activities implemented to improve the department.
4. Participates in the evaluation of orientation policies and procedures and recommends revisions to Supervisor.
5. Participates in the evaluation of inservice education programs.
6. Evaluates achievement or lack of achievement of desired outcomes.
   6.1 Data are collected concerning the patient's health status.
   6.2 Data are compared to the specific desired outcomes.
   6.3 Includes the patient in evaluation of the achievement of desired outcomes.
7. From evaluation of achievement or lack of achievement of desired outcomes, reassesses and revises the nursing care plan.

   From evaluation:
   7.1 Reassesses the patient problems.
   7.2 Reassesses desired outcomes to determine if appropriate, realistic, and in correct priority.
   7.3 Reassesses nursing prescriptions to determine if appropriate, realistic, and stated accurately.
   7.4 Reassesses nursing actions for effectiveness in achieving desired outcomes.

   From reassessment:
   7.5 Determines new patient present/potential problems.
   7.6 From new patient problems, formulates and revises desired outcomes.
   7.7 Revises nursing prescriptions.
   7.8 Implements new actions in order to carry out revised prescriptions.
   7.9 Continually evaluates desired outcomes for achievement or lack of achievement.
   7.10 Continually evaluates and revises the nursing care plan according to changes in the patient's health status.

SURGICAL REGISTERED NURSE: PERFORMANCE EVALUATION

Name ————————————— Employment Date —————————

Rating Period ———————————— To —————————————

Department ————————————— Job Title —————————————

Instructions: Using the following rating scale, indicate the quality of performance by placing the appropriate letter on the line to the left of the item.

U*– Unsatisfactory (does not meet job requirements)
S – Satisfactory (meets job requirements)
A – Above average (exceeds job requirements)
E* – Exceptional performance

I. *Assessment:*

——— 1. Assesses the number and level of personnel needed to provide quality patient care in the department and collaborates with the Supervisor in adjusting staffing and assignments.

———————————————————————————

———————————————————————————

——— 2. Participates in the assessment of functions and activities in Operating Room/Recovery Room as they relate to other departments.

———————————————————————————

———————————————————————————

——— 3. Assesses the delivery of nursing care in the department and identifies problems and any need for improvements.

———————————————————————————

———————————————————————————

——— 4. Assesses the health status of all patients, as outlined in the Standards of Surgical Nursing Practice and under hospital policy, prior to the surgical procedure.
   4.1 Completes a patient history and physical pertinent to the surgical procedure but is not limited to:
   a. Site preparation for surgical procedure
   b. Patterns of communication
   c. Preferred nickname
   d. Nutritional status

———————————————

*The evaluator is expected to comment on all items rated "U" or "E."

    e. Emotional status

    f. Patterns of coping

    g. Patient's concerns during or dealing with surgical procedure

    h. Patient's understanding of surgical procedure

    i. Patient's expected outcomes from surgical procedure

    j. Patient's perception of body image

    k. Patient's understanding of behaviors expected following surgical procedure

4.2 Collects data from patient, family and significant others, and health care providers.

4.3 Collects data by interview, observation, inspection, auscultation, and palpation.

4.4 Assesses and interprets reports and records, verbalizes pertinent information among health team members:

    a. Accurate identification of patient

    b. Complete consent form

    c. Preanethesia evaluation

    d. Confirmation of surgical site

    e. Vital signs (and time)

    f. Preoperative medications (and time)

    g. CBC, U/A, EKG and CXR, and other lab or x-ray reports

    h. Last oral intake

    i. Time of last voiding

    j. Other pertinent reports

4.5 Organizes assessment data so that they are accurate, complete, and accessible, and so that they remain confidential.

4.6 Communicates assessment data in an orderly fashion among the health team preoperatively, intraoperatively, and postoperatively and records and revises appropriately.

II. *Planning:*

_____ 1. Serves on hospital committees as requested.

_____

_____

_____ 2. Participates in developing, reviewing, and revising policies and procedures as directed by Supervisor.

_____

_____

_____ 3. Plans and develops self-objectives.

_____

_____

_____ 4. Plans ways to solve problems and to make improvements in the department in collaboration with the Supervisor.

_____

_____

_____ 5. Completes a written care plan for assigned patients. Plans the care for individual patients as well as directs and supervises others in the planning of patients' care.
   5.1 Identifies the patient's present/potential problems from the patient assessment:
       a. Patient's health status is determined,
       b. Health status is compared to the norms,
       c. Problems are given priority according to impact upon the patient's health status.

_____

_____

   5.2 Formulates desired outcomes, specific to the patient problems and established norms.

_____

_____

   5.3 Ensures that desired outcomes are mutually agreed upon by the patient and nurse and are:
       a. Specific
       b. Measurable within a certain time frame
       c. Consistent with other health providers' expectations

_____

_____

_____ 6. Incorporates postoperative care into expected outcomes by preoperative teaching, including but not limited to:

6.1 Explanation of surgical procedure.

_____

_____

6.2 Medication—preoperative medications, pain medications, and postoperative medications.

_____

_____

6.3 Diet (i.e., NPO) plan for progression following the procedure.

_____

_____

6.4 Exercise/activity: cough, turn and deep-breathing techniques, ambulation, and other expected behaviors or limitations.

_____

_____

6.5 Explanation of any extraneous equipment necessary following the procedure, (i.e., IV, nasogastric tube, Foley catheter, hemovac drain).

_____

_____

6.6 Self-care techniques and materials.

_____

_____

6.7 Available support systems, health information and resources that will enable the patient to understand and accept necessary modifications in body image and/or life-style.

_____

_____

III. _Implementation:_

_____ 1. Implements activities necessary to meeting self-objectives.

_____

_____

_____ 2. Participates in implementing planned changes and activities to improve the department.

_____

_____

_____ 3. Holds self and staff accountable for the delivery of quality nursing care.

_____

_____

_____ 4. Promotes harmonious relationships and favorable attitudes among the health care team.

_____

_____

_____ 5. Supports and adheres to nursing service and administrative policies and procedures.

_____

_____

_____ 6. Assists with orientation of new employees.

_____

_____

_____ 7. Acts rapidly and effectively, manages self, patients, and other employees during any emergency situation.

_____

_____

_____ 8. Attends required inservice education programs.

_____

_____

_____ 9. Formulates nursing prescriptions that delineate actions to be taken.
Prescribed actions:
9.1 Are specific to the patient's problems and desired outcomes.

_____

9.2 Are based on scientific knowledge.

_____

9.3 Are based on principles of psychosocial interactions.

_____

9.4 Are based on principles of preoperative patient teaching.

_____

_____

9.5 Include human, material, and community resources.

___

9.6 Include keeping patient knowledgeable of health status and total health care plan.

___

_____ 10. Implements the actions delineated in the nursing prescriptions. Actions implemented:
10.1 Actively involve the patient and family.

___

10.2 Are based on current scientific knowledge.

___

10.3 Are flexible and individualized for each patient.

___

10.4 Provide patient privacy and dignity.

___

10.5 Incorporate principles of safety.

___

10.6 Incorporate principles of infection control.

___

10.7 Reflect environmental factors affecting patient's health.

___

_____ 11. Demonstrates knowledge of and skill in exercising all Operating Room/Recovery Room procedures.

___

_____ 12. Demonstrates knowledge of location, care, and use of all equipment and supplies pertaining to Operating Room/Recovery Room.

___

_____ 13. Demonstrates knowledge of sterile/aseptic technique and recognizes and corrects any breaks in this technique.

_____

_____

_____ 14. Is always available and accessible when on duty or on call.

_____

_____

_____ 15. Conforms to hopsital dress code.

_____

_____

_____ 16. Is rarely sick or absent from work due to health.

_____

_____

_____ 17. Is prompt.

_____

_____

IV. *Evaluation:*

_____ 1. Evaluates Operating Room/Recovery Room policies and procedures and recommends the need for revision as assigned by Supervisor.

_____

_____

_____ 2. Evaluates self-objectives and determines need for revisions and new objectives.

_____

_____

_____ 3. Evaluates the efectiveness of problem-solving techniques and the activities implemented to improve the department.

_____

_____

_____ 4. Participates in the evaluation of orientation policies and procedures and recommends revisions to Supervisor.

_____

_____

_____ 5. Participates in the evaluation of inservice education programs.

_____

_____

_____ 6. Evaluates achievement or lack of achievement of desired outcomes.

6.1 Data are collected concerning the patient's health status.

_____

_____

6.2 Data are compared to the specific desired outcomes.

_____

_____

6.3 Includes the patient in evaluation of the achievement of desired outcomes.

_____

_____

_____ 7. From evaluation of achievement or lack of achievement of desired outcomes, reassesses and revises the nursing care plan.

From evaluation:
7.1 Reassesses the patient problems.

_____

_____

7.2 Reassesses desired outcomes to determine if appropriate, realistic, and in correct priority.

_____

_____

7.3 Reassesses nursing prescriptions to determine if appropriate, realistic, and stated accurately.

_____

_____

7.4 Reassesses nursing actions for effectiveness in achieving desired outcomes.

_____

_____

From reassessment:
7.5 Determines new patient present/potential problems.

_____

_____

7.6 From new patient problems formulates and revises desired outcomes.

_____

_____

7.7   Revises nursing prescriptions.

_____

_____

7.8   Implements new actions in order to carry out revised prescriptions.

_____

_____

7.9   Continually evaluates desired outcomes for achievement or lack of achievement.

_____

_____

7.10   Continually evaluates and revises the nursing care plan according to changes in the patient's health status.

_____

_____

SURGICAL REGISTERED NURSE: SCORING PROCEDURE

Instructions: Total the number of each item and multiply times the appropriate number. Add these totals to make the score.

U _____ × 0 = _____

S _____ × 1 = _____

A _____ × 2 = _____

E _____ × 3 = _____   _____ Total Score

Compare total score to the following scale to determine rank:

U	S	A	E
0 to 30	31 to 53	54 to 81	82 to 102

Overall Performance Review Score _____.

ALL ITEMS IN THE FOLLOWING SECTION MUST BE COMPLETED:

A. Interviewer's comments on overall review _____

_____

_____

B. Additional suggestions for overall work improvement and goals for next evaluation _____

_____

_____

C. Self-objectives _____

_____

_____

_____   _____
Date   Employee's signature

_____   _____
Date   Interviewer's signature

_____   _____
Date   Director of Nursing

SURGICAL LICENSED PRACTICAL NURSE: JOB DESCRIPTION

Position Requirements: Graduate from an accredited school for Licensed Practical Nurses with current licensure in the State of Alabama. Membership in LPN Association desired but not required. Participates in educational conferences and updates and maintains professional knowledge and skills related to areas of practice.

Position Accountable for: All nursing care behaviors described in the Surgical Licensed Practical Nurse job description.

Position Accountable to: Registered Nurse in charge of unit, Supervisor, Director of Nursing, and patient and family.

Position Summary: Performs the functions of a Licensed Practical Nurse in assessing, planning, implementing, and evaluating all assigned patient care in collaboration with a Registered Nurse. Is accountable for all patient care she gives during a shift. Is responsible for adhering to Surgical Standards of Nursing Practice, for managing supplies and equipment with the direction of the Registered Nurse in charge, and for promoting teamwork with physicians and personnel of other departments.

I. *Assessment*

1. Assesses nursing care given by self; identifies problems and/or need for improvement and communicates this information to the Supervisor.

2. Participates in patient assessment according to Surgical Nursing Standards of Practice, as directed by Registered Nurse.

   2.1 Utilizes data collected from the patient, family and significant others, health care providers, individuals, and/or agencies in the community.

   2.2 Utilizes data collected by interview, observation, inspection, auscultation, palpation, and reports and records.

   2.3 Organizes assessment data so that they are accurate, complete, and accessible, and so that they remain confidential.

   2.4 Communicates assessment data in an orderly fashion by recording, updating, and revising as appropriate. Communicates pertinent information on a continual basis to the Registered Nurse in charge.

3. Assesses patient charts preoperatively for completeness, as outlined in hospital policies.

4. Assesses patient for proper identification and verifies operative site—as well as proper preoperative skin preparation.

II. *Planning*
1. Reviews and revises Operating Room/Recovery Room policies and procedures when requested.
2. Plans and develops self-objectives with Supervisor, in conjunction with performance evaluation.
3. Suggests ways to solve problems and make improvements in the department.
4. In collaboration with the Registered Nurse contributes to the formulation of patient care plans:
    4.1 Identifies patient problems.
    4.2 Formulates desired outcomes.
    4.3 Communicates the above to the Registered Nurse.

III. *Implementation*
1. Implements activities necessary to meeting self-objectives.
2. Cooperates with the Registered Nurse in implementing planned changes and activities to improve nursing care in the department.
3. Promotes harmonious relationships and favorable attitudes among the health care team.
4. Supports and adheres to nursing service and administrative policies and procedures.
5. Assists with orientation of new employees.
6. Is knowledgeable of equipment and assists with management of assigned patients during emergencies.
7. Attends required inservice education programs.
8. Participates with Registered Nurse in the implementation of assigned patient's plan of care.
9. Documents nursing actions implemented, and effectiveness of implementation, in the nurses' notes in a continuous manner.
10. Demonstrates knowledge of and skill in exercising all Operating Room/Recovery Room procedures.
11. Demonstrates knowledge of location, care, and use of all equipment/supplies pertaining to Operating Room/Recovery Room.
12. Demonstrates knowledge of sterile/aseptic technique and recognizes and corrects any breaks in this technique.
13. Is always available and accessible when on duty or on call.
14. Conforms to hospital dress code.
15. Is rarely sick or absent from work due to health.
16. Is prompt.

IV. *Evaluation*
1. Evaluates the nursing care she gives.
2. Evaluates self-objectives and determines need for new objectives.
3. Evaluates the effectiveness of problem-solving techniques and activities implemented to improve nursing care in the department.

4. Evaluates Licensed Practical Nurse orientation policies and procedures and recommends revisions.
5. Participates in the evaluation of inservice education programs.
6. Participates with the Registered Nurse in the evaluation and revision of assigned patient's plan of care.

SURGICAL LICENSED PRACTICAL NURSE: PERFORMANCE EVALUATION

Name _____ Employment Date _____

Rating Period _____ To _____

Department _____ Job Title _____

Instructions: Using the following rating scale, indicate the quality of performance by placing the appropriate letter on the line to the left of the item.

U* – Unsatisfactory (does not meet job requirements)
S – Satisfactory (meets job requirements)
A – Above average (exceeds job requirements)
E* – Exceptional performance

I. *Assessment:*

_____ 1. Assesses nursing care given by self and identifies problems and/or need for improvement and communicates this information to the Supervisor.

_____

_____

_____ 2. Participates in patient assessment according to Surgical Nursing Standards of Practice, as directed by Registered Nurse.
  2.1 Utilizes data collected from the patient, family and significant others, health care providers, individuals, and/or agencies in the community.

_____

_____

  2.2 Utilizes data collected by interview, observation, inspection, auscultation, palpation, and reports and records.

_____

_____

  2.3 Organizes assessment data so that they are accurate, complete, and accessible, and so that they remain confidential.

_____

_____

_____

*The evaluator is expected to comment on all items rated "U" or "E."

    2.4 Communicates assessment data in an orderly fashion by recording, updating, and revising as appropriate. Communicates pertinent information on a continual basis to the Registered Nurse in charge.

_____ 3. Assesses patient charts preoperatively for completeness, as outlined in hospital policies.

_____ 4. Assesses patient for proper identification and verifying operative site, as well as proper preoperative skin preparation.

II. *Planning:*

_____ 1. Reviews and revises Operating Room/Recovery Room policies and procedures when requested.

_____ 2. Plans and develops self-objectives with Supervisor in conjunction with performance evaluation.

_____ 3. Suggests ways to solve problems and to make improvements in the department.

_____ 4. In collaboration with the Registered Nurse, contributes to the formulation of patient care plans:
    4.1 Identifies patient problems.

    4.2 Formulates desired outcomes.

    4.3 Communicates the above to the Registered Nurse.

III. *Implementation:*

———— 1. Implements activities necessary to meeting self-objectives.

_____

_____

———— 2. Cooperates with the Registered Nurse in implementing planned changes and activities to improve nursing care in the department.

_____

_____

———— 3. Promotes harmonious relationships and favorable attitudes among the health care team.

_____

_____

———— 4. Supports and adheres to nursing service and administrative policies and procedures.

_____

_____

———— 5. Assists with orientation of new employees.

_____

_____

———— 6. Is knowledgeable of equipment and assists with management of assigned patients during emergencies.

_____

_____

———— 7. Attends required inservice education programs.

_____

_____

———— 8. Participates with Registered Nurse in the implementation of assigned patient's plan of care.

_____

_____

———— 9. Documents nursing actions implemented, and effectiveness of implementation, in the nurses' notes in a continuous manner.

_____

_____

_____ 10. Demonstrates knowledge of and skill in exercising all Operating Room/Recovery Room procedures.

_____

_____

_____ 11. Demonstrates knowledge of location, care, and use of all equipment and supplies pertaining to Operating Room/Recovery Room.

_____

_____

_____ 12. Demonstrates knowledge of sterile/aseptic technique and recognizes and corrects any breaks in this technique.

_____

_____

_____ 13. Is always available and accessible when on duty or on call.

_____

_____

_____ 14. Conforms to hospital dress code.

_____

_____

_____ 15. Is rarely sick or absent from work due to health.

_____

_____

_____ 16. Is prompt.

_____

_____

IV. *Evaluation:*

_____ 1. Evaluates the nursing care she gives.

_____

_____

_____ 2. Evaluates self-objectives and determines need for new objectives.

_____

_____

_____ 3. Evaluates the effectiveness of problem-solving techniques and activities implemented to improve nursing care in the department.

_____

_____

_____ 4. Evaluates Licensed Practical Nurse orientation policies and procedures and recommends revisions.

_____

_____

_____ 5. Participates in the evaluation of inservice education programs.

_____

_____

_____ 6. Participates with the Registered Nurse in the evaluation and revision
of assigned patient's plan of care.

_____

_____

SURGICAL LICENSED PRACTICAL NURSE: SCORING PROCEDURE

Instructions: Total the number of each item and multiply times the appropriate number. Add these totals to make the score.

U _____ ×0= _____

S _____ ×1= _____

A _____ ×2= _____

E _____ ×3= _____   _____ Total Score

Compare total score to the following scale to determine rank:

U	S	A	E
0 to 26	27 to 47	48 to 71	72 to 90

Overall Performance Review Score _____.

ALL ITEMS IN THE FOLLOWING SECTION MUST BE COMPLETED:

A. Interviewer's comments on overall review _____

_____

_____

B. Additional suggestions for overall work improvement and goals for next evaluation _____

_____

_____

C. Self-objectives _____

_____

_____

_____

_____

_____ Date   _____ Employee's signature

_____ Date   _____ Interviewer's signature

_____ Date   _____ Director of Nursing

10
Emergency Nursing Practice

STANDARDS OF EMERGENCY NURSING PRACTICE

STANDARD I

Assessment is the identification and gathering of data concerning the health status of the patient. This process is complete and systematic as evidenced by:

1. *Assessment of the patient's immediate needs and prioritizing data according to this initial assessment.*
2. *A pertinent patient history:*
   a. *Patient interview:*
      Chief complaint
      History of present illness
      Allergies
      Medications
      Recent medical/surgical history
      Cultural, socioeconomic, and environmental conditions pertinent to health care
      Pertinent family history
      Available and accessible human, community, and material resources
3. *Assessment of alterations or deficits in body systems/responses:*
   Mental
   Emotional
   Nutritional
   Personal habits
   Activity level
   Hygiene/grooming
   Coping mechanism
   Communication
   Interaction
   Vital signs
   Head, eye, ear, nose, and throat
   Cardiovascular
   Respiratory
   Integumentary
   Gastrointestinal
   Musculoskeletal
   Genitourinary
   Fluid and electrolyte
4. *Assessment of pain:*
   Location
   Quality
   Quantity
   Onset
   Duration
   Chronology

Associated manifestations
Alleviating mechanisms

5. *Assessment of perceptions and knowledge level pertinent to health care:*
   Concerns related to health status/care
   Knowledge of disease process/alteration in health status
   Understanding of health care or reasons for hospitalization
   Expected outcome from health care

6. *The collection of data from available sources:*
   Patient, family/significant others
   Health care providers
   Consultation

7. *The collection of data by scientific methodology:*
   Interview
   Observation
   Inspection
   Auscultation
   Palpation

8. *Collection of data by the interpretation/assessment and communication of reports and records:*
   Electrocardiogram
   Radiology studies
   Hematology studies
   Chemistry studies
   Coagulation studies
   Arterial blood gases
   Urinalysis
   Previous records

9. *The organization of data in a systematic arrangement:* The arrangement provides:
   Accurate collection
   Complete collection
   Accessibility
   Confidentiality

10. *The communication of data in an orderly fashion:*
    Data are recorded.
    Data are updated.
    Data are communicated verbally among health team.
    Data are communicated to appropriate agencies when necessary.

STANDARD II

Nursing care planning consists of determining patient problems and desired outcomes. Planning involves preparing the patient for home care. This is evidenced by:

1. *The identification of present/potential patient problems, from the patient assessment:* Data are grouped into meaningful arrangement, based upon scientific knowledge.

Patient's health status is determined.

Patient's health status is compared to the norms.

Present and potential problems are identified.

Problems are given priority according to impact upon the patient's health status.

2. *The formulation of desired outcomes:*

Patient (family, significant other) and nurse mutually agree upon the patient's present/potential health problems.

Patient and nurse mutually agree upon desired outcomes.

Desired outcomes are congruent with the patient problems and established norms.

Desired outcomes are specific.

Desired outcomes are measurable.

Desired outcomes are consistent with other health providers' expectations.

Desired outcomes are established to restore patient's optimal functioning capabilities.

3. *The incorporation of home health care into desired outcomes. This involves teaching:*

Disease process/alteration in health status

Expected outcomes from health care

Complications and prevention

Specific signs and symptoms that dictate notifying health team

Medication

Diet

Exercise/activity

Self-care techniques and materials

Available support systems and resources

Follow-up care

STANDARD III

The plan of care is implemented in order to achieve the desired outcome. This is evidenced by:

1. *The formulation of nursing prescriptions that delineate actions to be taken. Prescribed actions:*

Are given priority according to desired outcomes, and to expedite implementation.

Are specific to identified patient problems and desired outcomes.

Are based on current scientific knowledge.

Incorporate principles of patient teaching.

Incorporate principles of psychosocial interactions.

Incorporate environmental factors influencing the patient's health.

Include human, material, and community resources and support systems.

Direct achieving optimal bio-psycho-social status.

Include keeping patient and family/significant other knowledgeable of health status and total health care plan.

2. *The implementation of actions delineated in the nursing prescriptions. Actions implemented:*

Actively involve the patient and family/significant other.
Are consistent with the nursing prescriptions.
Are based upon current scientific knowledge.
Are flexible and individualized for each patient.
Include principles of safety.
Include principles of infection control.
Include principles of noise and traffic control.
Provide for patient privacy and dignity.
Reflect "A Patient's Bill of Rights."

STANDARD IV

Outcomes of Nursing Actions are evaluated for further assessment and planning. This is evidenced by:

1. *Evaluating the achievement of desired outcomes:*
   Data are collected concerning the patient's health status.
   Data are compared to the specific desired outcomes.
   The patient, family/significant other, and nurse evaluate the achievement of desired outcomes.
2. *Reassessment of the nursing care plan:*
   Outcome of nursing actions direct the reassessment of identified patient problems.
   Outcome of nursing actions direct assessment of desired outcomes (assess the desired outcome to determine if appropriate, realistic, and in correct priority).
   Outcome of nursing actions direct reassessment of nursing prescriptions (assess the nursing prescriptions to determine if appropriate, realistic, and stated accurately).
   Nursing actions are assessed for effectiveness in achieving desired outcomes.
3. *Further planning as directed by the reassessment:*
   Reassessment determines new patient present/potential problems.
   New patient problems direct the formulation and revision of desired outcomes.
   Revised desired outcomes direct the revising of nursing prescriptions.
   Revised prescriptions direct new actions to be implemented toward desired outcomes.
   Desired outcomes are continually evaluated and revised according to changes in the patient's health status.

EMERGENCY SUPERVISOR: JOB DESCRIPTION

Position Requirements:	Graduate from an accredited school of nursing with current licensure as a registered nurse in the State of Alabama. At least 1 year clinical experience in Emergency Department with Supervisory training.
Professional Requirements:	Pursues programs of continuing education consistent with requirements of the Alabama Nurses' Association. Participates in educational conferences and updates and maintains professional knowledge and skills related to the management areas of responsibility.
Position Accountable for:	All nursing care behaviors described in the Emergency Department Supervisor job description.
Position Accountable to:	Director of Nursing Service, patient, and family.
Position Summary:	Is responsible for meeting the Joint Commission Standards of Patient Care and the established Standards of Emergency Nursing Practice, for managing all personnel, supplies, and equipment in the Emergency Department, and for promoting teamwork with physicians and personnel of other departments. Directs and ensures that all patients in the Emergency Department are assessed, and their care is planned, implemented, and evaluated. Is accountable on a 24-hour basis.

I. *Assessment*
1. Assesses the number and level of personnel needed to provide quality patient care and adjusts staffing and assignments appropriately.
2. Assesses the overall operation of the Emergency Department on a continual basis and identifies problem areas and need for improvement in the delivery of patient care.
3. Ensures that the health status of all patients is assessed upon arrival in the Emergency Room, as outlined in the Nursing Standards. Ensures that:
   3.1 The patient's needs are assessed and data are prioritized accordingly.
   3.2 A pertinent patient history is obtained.
   3.3 A patient assessment is completed including:
      a. assessment of alterations or deficits in body systems/responses,
      b. assessment of pain associated with any alterations or deficits,

      c. patient's perceptions,

      d. knowledge level pertinent to health care.

3.4 Data are collected from patient, family, significant others, and health care providers, and by consultation with appropriate personnel.

3.5 Data are collected by interview, observation, inspection, auscultation, and palpation.

3.6 All data collected from reports and records are assessed and interpreted appropriately.

3.7 Assessment data are organized so that they are accurate, complete, and accessible, and so that they remain confidential.

3.8 Assessment data are communicated in an orderly fashion by recording, updating, and verbalizing pertinent information to health team members and to appropriate agencies.

II. *Planning*

1. Develops, reviews, and revises all policies and procedures for the Emergency Department with approval of the Director of Nursing.

2. Plans and develops self-objectives.

3. Plans ways to solve problems and make improvements in the delivery of patient care.

4. Ensures that an individualized care plan is formulated for all patients seen in the Emergency Department. Ensures that:

    4.1 The patient's present/potential problems are identified from the patient's assessment.

      a. data are based upon current scientific knowledge,

      b. patient's health status is determined,

      c. patient's health status is compared to the norm,

      d. problems are given priority according to impact upon the patient's health status.

    4.2 Desired outcomes are formulated specific to the patient's problems and established norms.

    4.3 Established desired outcomes are mutually agreed upon by the nurse, patient, family and significant others and are (a) measurable, (b) consistent with other health care providers' expectations, and (c) established to restore patient's optimal functioning capabilities.

    4.4 Home health care is incorporated into patient's desired outcomes. This includes but is not limited to teaching concerning:

      a. disease process/alterations in health status

      b. desired outcomes from health care

      c. complications and prevention

      d. specific signs and symptoms that dictate notifying the health team

      e. medication

      f. diet

      g. exercise/activity

      h. self-care techniques and materials

      i. available support systems and resources

      j. follow-up care

III. *Implementation*

 1. Implements activities necessary to meeting self-objectives.
 2. From assessments and identification of problems and needs, implements planned changes and activities to improve Emergency Department in collaboration with the Director of Nursing.
 3. Promotes the achievement of Emergency Department objectives.
 4. Ensures that Standards of Emergency Nursing Practice are implemented and monitors standards as necessary.
 5. Holds self and staff accountable for the delivery of quality nursing care.
 6. Ensures that department is at all times clean and organized and supplies are restocked as necessary.
 7. Acts rapidly and effectively, follows hospital policies and procedures, and utilizes principles of management in any emergency situation.
 8. Promotes harmonious relationships and favorable attitudes among the health care team.
 9. Interprets, supports, and recommends administrative and nursing service policies and procedures for employees and ensures compliance. Applies knowledge and skills of management.
10. Assists with orientation of new employees.
11. Keeps the Director of Nursing Service informed on reportable situations and needs.
12. Attends required inservice education programs.
13. Implements and directs personnel in implementing the patient's plan of care.
14. Ensures that nursing prescriptions are formulated that delineate actions to be taken. Ensures that prescribed actions:
    14.1 Are given priority according to desired outcomes.
    14.2 Are specific to the patient's problems and desired outcomes.
    14.3 Are based on current scientific knowledge.
    14.4 Incorporate principles of patient teaching.
    14.5 Incorporate principles of psychosocial interactions.
    14.6 Incorporate environmental factors influencing patient's health.
    14.7 Include human, material, and community resources and support systems.
    14.8 Direct achievement of optimal bio-psycho-social status.
    14.9 Include keeping the patient, family, and significant others aware of the total health care plan.
15. Ensures that actions implemented are delineated in the nursing prescriptions. Actions implemented:
    15.1 Actively involve the patient, family, and significant others.
    15.2 Are consistent with the nursing prescriptions.
    15.3 Are based upon current scientific knowledge.
    15.4 Are flexible and individualized for each patient.
    15.5 Include principles of safety.
    15.6 Include principles of infection control.

15.7 Provide for patient privacy and dignity.

15.8 Reflect "A Patient's Bill of Rights."

16. Serves as consultant in technical and professional matters for personnel.

17. Participates and contributes to a unified Quality Assurance Program.

18. Participates in the provision of inservice education programs, related to Emergency Nursing.

19. Conforms to hospital dress code.

20. Is rarely sick or absent from work due to health.

21. Is prompt and attends report.

22. Serves on hospital committees as requested.

IV. *Evaluation*

1. Continually evaluates the Emergency Standards of Nursing Practice by assessing patients, reviewing charts, interviewing and observing, participating in Quality Assurance activities, and by employing other means of evaluation. Revises standards as appropriate in collaboration with Director of Nursing.

2. Evaluates policies and procedures and revises as necessary.

3. Evaluates self-objectives and determines need for revision and new objectives.

4. Evaluates activities to improve operation of the department and evaluates the effectiveness of problem-solving techniques and approaches.

5. Evaluates the performance of nursing service personnel in the department.

6. Evaluates the achievement of Emergency Department objectives in collaboration with Director of Nursing Service.

7. Evaluates emergencies and any hospital disaster and recommends revisions in policies and procedures and/or need for improvement in employee performance.

8. Evaluates orientation policies and procedures and recommends revisions.

9. Evaluates inservice education programs.

10. Ensures that desired outcomes are evaluated for achievement or lack of achievement.

    10.1 Data are collected concerning the patient's health status.

    10.2 Data are compared to the specific desired outcomes.

    10.3 The patient and nurse evaluate the achievement of desired outcomes.

11. Ensures that the nursing care plan is reassessed and revised from the evaluation of achievement or lack of achievement of desired outcomes.

    From evaluation:

    11.1 Reassesses the patient's problems.

    11.2 Reassesses desired outcomes to determine if appropriate, realistic, and in correct priority.

11.3   Reassesses nursing prescriptions to determine if appropriate, realistic, and stated accurately.

11.4   Reassessment of nursing actions for effectiveness in achieving desired outcomes.

From reassessment:

11.5   Determines new patient present/potential problems.

11.6   From new patient problems, formulates and revises desired outcomes.

11.7   Revises nursing prescriptions.

11.8   Implements new actions in order to carry out revised prescriptions.

11.9   Continually evaluates nursing actions and desired outcomes for achievement or lack of achievement.

11.10 Continually evaluates and revises the nursing care plan according to changes in the patient's health status.

EMERGENCY SUPERVISOR: PERFORMANCE EVALUATION

Name _____ Employment Date _____

Rating Period _____ To _____

Department _____ Job Title _____

Instructions: Using the following rating scale, indicate the quality of performance by placing the appropriate letter on the line to the left of the item.

U* – Unsatisfactory (does not meet job requirements)
S – Satisfactory (meets job requirements)
A – Above average (exceeds job requirements)
E* – Exceptional performance

I. *Assessment:*

_____ 1. Assesses the number and level of personnel needed to provide quality patient care and adjusts staffing and assignments appropriately.

_____ 2. Assesses the overall operation of the Emergency Department on a continual basis and identifies problem areas and need for improvement in the delivery of patient care.

_____ 3. Ensures that the health status of all patients is assessed upon arrival in the Emergency Room, as outlined in the Nursing Standards. Ensures that:
3.1 The patient's needs are assessed and data are prioritized accordingly.

3.2 A pertinent patient history is obtained.

3.3 A patient assessment is completed, including:
a. Assessment of alterations or deficits in body systems/responses,

*The evaluator is expected to comment on all items rated "U" or "E."

207

  b. Assessment of pain associated with any alterations or deficits,
  c. Patient's perceptions,
  d. Knowledge level pertinent to health care.

_____

3.4 Data are collected from patient, family, significant others, health
care providers, and by consultation with appropriate personnel.

_____

3.5 Data are collected by interview, observation, inspection, auscultation, and palpation.

_____

3.6 All data collected from reports and records are assessed and
interpreted appropriately.

_____

3.7 Assessment data are organized so that they are accurate, complete, and accessible, and so that they remain confidential.

_____

3.8 Assessment data are communicated in an orderly fashion by
recording, updating, and verbalizing pertinent information to
health team members and to appropriate agencies.

_____

_____

II. *Planning:*

_____ 1. Develops, reviews, and revises all policies and procedures for the
Emergency Department with approval of the Director of Nursing.

_____

_____ 2. Plans and develops self-objectives.

_____

_____ 3. Plans ways to solve problems and make improvements in the delivery
of patient care.

_____

_____

_____ 4. Ensures that an individualized care plan is formulated for all patients seen in the Emergency Department. Ensures that:

4.1 The patient's present/potential problems are identified from the
patient's assessment.
   a. Data are based upon current scientific knowledge,
   b. Patient's health status is determined,
   c. Patient's health status is compared to the norm,
   d. Problems are given priority according to impact upon the
   patient's health status.

4.2 Desired outcomes are formulated specific to the patient's problems and established norms.

4.3 Established desired outcomes are mutually agreed upon by the
nurse, patient, family, and significant others and are:
   a. Measurable
   b. Consistent with other health care providers' expectations
   c. Established to restore patient's optimal functioning capabilities

4.4 Home health care is incorporated into patient's desired outcomes. This includes but is not limited to teaching concerning:
   a. Disease process/alterations in health status
   b. Desired outcomes from health care
   c. Complications and prevention
   d. Specific signs and symptoms that dictate notifying the health
   team
   e. Medication
   f. Diet
   g. Exercise/activity
   h. Self-care techniques and materials
   i. Available support systems and resources
   j. Follow-up care

III. _Implementation:_

_____ 1. Implements activities necessary to meeting self-objectives.

_____ 2. From assessments and identification of problems and needs, implements planned changes and activities to improve Emergency Department in collaboration with the Director of Nursing.

_____ 3. Promotes the achievement of Emergency Department objectives.

_____ 4. Ensures that Standards of Emergency Nursing Practice are implemented; monitors standards as necessary.

_____ 5. Holds self and staff accountable for the delivery of quality nursing care.

_____ 6. Ensures that department is at all times clean and organized and supplies are restocked as necessary.

_____ 7. Acts rapidly and effectively, follows hospital policies and procedures, and utilizes principles of management in any emergency situation.

_____ 8. Promotes harmonious relationships and favorable attitudes among the health care team.

_____ 9. Interprets, supports, and recommends administrative and nursing service policies and procedures for employees and ensures compliance. Applies knowledge and skills of management.

_____ 10. Assists with orientation of new employees.

_____ 11. Keeps the Director of Nursing Service informed on reportable situations and needs.

_____ 12. Attends required inservice education programs.

_____ 13. Implements and directs personnel in implementing the patient's plan of care.

_____ 14. Ensures that nursing prescriptions are fomulated that delineate actions to be taken. Ensures that prescribed actions:
14.1 Are given priority according to desired outcomes.

14.2 Are specific to the patient's problems and desired outcomes.

14.3 Are based on current scientific knowledge.

14.4 Incorporate principles of patient teaching.

14.5 Incorporate principles of psychosocial interactions.

14.6 Incorporate environmental factors influencing patient's health.

14.7 Include human, material, and community resources and support systems.

14.8 Direct achievement of optimal bio-psycho-social status.

14.9 Include keeping the patient, family, and significant others aware of the total health care plan.

_____

_____

_____ 15. Ensures that actions implemented are delineated in the nursing prescriptions. Actions implemented:
15.1 Actively involve the patient, family, and significant others.

_____

15.2 Are consistent with the nursing prescriptions.

_____

15.3 Are based upon current scientific knowledge.

_____

15.4 Are flexible and individualized for each patient.

_____

15.5 Include principles of safety.

_____

15.6 Include principles of infection control.

_____

15.7 Provide for patient privacy and dignity.

_____

15.8 Reflect "A Patient's Bill of Rights."

_____

_____ 16. Serves as consultant in technical and professional matters for personnel.

_____

_____ 17. Participates and contributes to a unified Quality Assurance Program.

_____

_____

_____ 18. Participates in the provision of inservice education programs related to Emergency Nursing.

_____

_____

_____ 19. Conforms to hospital dress code.

_____

_____

_____ 20. Is rarely sick or absent from work due to health.

_____

_____

_____ 21. Is prompt and attends report.

_____

_____

_____ 22. Serves on hospital committees as requested.

_____

_____

IV. *Evaluation:*

_____ 1. Continually evaluates the Emergency Standards of Nursing Practice by assessing patients, reviewing charts, interviewing and observing, participating in Quality Assurance activities, and by employing other means of evaluation. Revises standards as appropriate in collaboration with Director of Nursing.

_____

_____

_____ 2. Evaluates policies and procedures and revises as necessary.

_____

_____

_____ 3. Evaluates self-objectives and determines need for revision and new objectives.

_____

_____

_____ 4. Evaluates activities to improve operation of the department and evaluates the effectiveness of problem-solving techniques and approaches.

_____

_____

_____ 5. Evaluates the performance of nursing service personnel in the department.

_____

_____

_____ 6. Evaluates the achievement of Emergency Department objectives in collaboration with Director of Nursing Service.

_____

_____

_____ 7. Evaluates emergencies and any hospital disaster and recommends revisions in policies and procedures and/or need for improvement in employee performance.

_____

_____

_____ 8. Evaluates orientation policies and procedures and recommends revisions.

_____

_____

_____ 9. Evaluates inservice education programs.

_____

_____

_____ 10. Ensures that desired outcomes are evaluated for achievement or lack of achievement.
10.1 Data are collected concerning the patient's health status.

_____

10.2 Data are compared to the specific desired outcomes.

_____

10.3 The patient and nurse evaluate the achievement of desired outcomes.

_____

_____

_____ 11. Ensures that the nursing care plan is reassessed and revised from the evaluation of achievement or lack of achievement of desired outcomes.

From evaluation:
11.1   Reassesses the patient's problems.

_____

_____

11.2 Reassesses desired outcomes to determine if appropriate, realistic, and in correct priority.

11.3 Reassesses nursing prescriptions to determine if appropriate, realistic, and stated accurately.

11.4 Reassessment of nursing actions for effectiveness in achieving desired outcomes.

From reassessment:

11.5 Determines new patient present/potential problems.

11.6 From new patient problems, formulates and revises desired outcomes.

11.7 Revises nursing prescriptions.

11.8 Implements new actions in order to carry out revised prescriptions.

11.9 Continually evaluates nursing actions and desired outcomes for achievement or lack of achievement.

11.10 Continually evaluates and revises the nursing care plan according to changes in the patient's health status.

EMERGENCY SUPERVISOR: SCORING PROCEDURE

Instructions: Total the number of each item and multiply times the appropriate number. Add these totals to make the score.

U _____ × 0 = _____

S _____ × 1 = _____

A _____ × 2 = _____

E _____ × 3 = _____   _____ Total Score

Compare total score to the following scale to determine rank:

U	S	A	E
0 to 35	36 to 63	64 to 95	96 to 120

Overall Performance Review Score _____.

ALL ITEMS IN THE FOLLOWING SECTION MUST BE COMPLETED:

A. Interviewer's comments on overall review _____

_____

_____

B. Additional suggestions for overall work improvement and goals for next evaluation _____

_____

_____

C. Self-objectives _____

_____

_____

_____

_____   _____
Date   Employee's signature

_____   _____
Date   Interviewer's signature

_____   _____
Date   Director of Nursing

EMERGENCY REGISTERED NURSE: JOB DESCRIPTION

Position Requirements:

Graduate from an accredited school of nursing with current licensure as a registered nurse in the State of Alabama. At least 1 year clinical experience preferred; specific orientation for the Emergency Department.

Professional Requirements:

Pursues programs of continuing education consistent with requirements of the Alabama Nurses' Association. Participates in educational conferences and updates and maintains professional knowledge and skills related to the areas of responsibility.

Position Accountable for:

All nursing care behaviors described in the Emergency Department Registered Nurse job description.

Position Accountable to:

Emergency Department Supervisor, Director of Nursing Service, patient, and family.

Position Summary:

Assesses, plans, implements, and evaluates the care of patients in the Emergency Department. Is responsible for managing all assigned personnel, supplies, and equipment in the Emergency Department and for promoting teamwork with physicians and personnel of other departments.

I. *Assessment*
1. Assesses the number and level of personnel needed to provide quality patient care and collaborates with the Supervisor in adjusting staffing.
2. Assesses the delivery of nursing care in the Emergency Department and identifies problems and any need for improvement.
3. Assesses the health status of all patients upon arrival in the Emergency Room as outlined in the nursing standards.
   3.1 Assesses the patient's immediate needs and data are prioritized accordingly.
   3.2 Obtains pertinent patient history.
   3.3 Completes a patient assessment that includes:
      a. assessment of alterations or deficits in body systems/responses,
      b. assessment of pain, associated with any alterations or deficits,
      c. patient's perceptions,
      d. knowledge level pertinent to health care.
   3.4 Collects data from patient, family, significant others, health care providers, and by consultation with appropriate personnel.

3.5 Collects data by interview, observation, inspection, auscultation, and palpation.

3.6 Interprets and assesses all data collected from reports and records.

3.7 Organizes assessment data so that they are accurate, complete, and accessible, and so that they remain confidential.

3.8 Communicates assessment data in an orderly fashion by recording, updating, and verbalizing pertinent information to health team members and to appropriate agencies.

II. *Planning*

1. Serves on hospital committees and helps to plan policies and procedures as directed by Supervisor.

2. Plans and develops self-objectives.

3. Plans ways to solve problems and to make improvements in the Emergency Department.

4. Formulates an individualized care plan for all patients seen in the Emergency Room.

   4.1 Identifies the patient's present/potential problems from the patient assessment.

   a. data are based on scientific knowledge,
   b. patient's health status is determined,
   c. patient's health status is compared to the norm,
   d. problems are given priority according to impact upon the patient's health status.

   4.2 Formulates desired outcomes, specific to the patient problems and established norms.

   4.3 Establishes desired outcomes that are mutually agreed upon by the nurse, patient, family, and significant others and are: (a) measurable, (b) consistent with other health care providers' expectations, and (c) established to restore patient's optimal functioning capabilities.

   4.4 Incorporates home health care into patient's desired outcomes. This includes but is not limited to teaching concerning:

   a. disease process/alteration in health status
   b. desired outcomes from health care
   c. complications and prevention
   d. specific signs and symptoms that dictate notifying the health team
   e. medications
   f. diet
   g. exercise/activity
   h. self-care techniques and materials
   i. available support systems and resources
   j. follow-up care

III. *Implementation*

1. Implements activities necessary to meeting self-objectives.

2. Participates in implementing planned changes and activities to improve the Emergency Department.

3. Holds self accountable for the delivery of quality nursing care.
4. Promotes harmonious relationships and favorable attitudes among the health care team.
5. Is knowledgeable of location, care, and operation of all Emergency Department equipment. This includes but is not limited to: Life Pack, sterile trays, crash cart contents, MAST trousers.
6. Directs Life Flight procedures.
7. Assists in keeping department clean and organized and restocks supplies as necessary.
8. Supports and adheres to administrative and nursing service policies and procedures.
9. Assists with orientation of new employees.
10. Acts rapidly, effectively, and manages self, patients, and other employees during any emergency situation.
11. Responds immediately to any emergency within the hospital.
12. Attends required inservice education programs.
13. Formulates nursing prescriptions that delineate actions to be taken. Prescribed actions:
    13.1 Are given priority according to desired outcomes.
    13.2 Are specific to the patient's problems and desired outcomes.
    13.3 Are based on current scientific knowledge.
    13.4 Are based on principles of patient teaching.
    13.5 Are based on principles of psychosocial interactions.
    13.6 Are based on environmental factors influencing patient's health.
    13.7 Include human, material, and community resources and support systems.
    13.8 Direct achievement of optimal bio-psycho-social status.
    13.9 Include keeping the patient, family, and significant others aware of the total health care plan.
14. Implements action delineated in the nursing prescriptions. Actions implemented:
    14.1 Actively involve the patient, family, and significant others.
    14.2 Are consistent with the nursing prescriptions.
    14.3 Are based upon current scientific knowledge.
    14.4 Are flexible and individualized for each patient.
    14.5 Include principles of safety.
    14.6 Include principles of infection control.
    14.7 Provide for patient privacy and dignity.
    14.8 Reflect a "Patient's Bill of Rights."
15. Conforms to hospital dress code.
16. Is rarely sick or absent from work due to health.
17. Is prompt and attends report.

IV. *Evaluation*
1. Evaluates self-objectives, revises and formulates new objectives.
2. Evaluates the effectiveness of problem-solving techniques and activities implemented to improve the Emergency Department.

3. Contributes to the performance evaluation of nursing personnel in the Emergency Department.
4. Participates in the evaluation of inservice education offerings.
5. Evaluates achievement or lack of achievement of desired outcomes.
   5.1 Data are collected concerning the patient's health status.
   5.2 Data are compared to the specific desired outcomes.
   5.3 Includes the patient's evaluation of the achievement of desired outcomes.
6. From evaluation of achievement or lack of achievement of desired outcomes, reassesses and revises the nursing care plan.

   From evaluation:
   6.1 Reassesses the patient problems.
   6.2 Reassesses desired outcomes to determine if appropriate, realistic, and in correct priority.
   6.3 Reassesses nursing prescriptions to determine if appropriate, realistic, and accurately stated.
   6.4 Reassesses nursing actions for effectiveness in achieving desired outcomes.

   From reassessment:
   6.5 Determines new patient present/potential problems.
   6.6 From new patient problems, formulates and revises desired outcomes.
   6.7 Revises nursing prescriptions.
   6.8 Implements new actions in order to carry out revised prescriptions.
   6.9 Continually evaluates desired outcomes for achievement or lack of achievement.
   6.10 Continually evaluates and revises the nursing care plan according to changes in the patient's health status.

EMERGENCY REGISTERED NURSE: PERFORMANCE EVALUATION

Name _____ Employment Date _____

Rating Period _____ To _____

Department _____ Job Title _____

Instructions: Using the following rating scale, indicate the quality of performance by placing the appropriate letter on the line to the left of the item.

U* – Unsatisfactory (does not meet job requirements)
S – Satisfactory (meets job requirements)
A – Above average (exceeds job requirements)
E* – Exceptional performance

I. *Assessment:*

_____ 1. Assesses the number and level of personnel needed to provide quality patient care and collaborates with the Supervisor in adjusting staffing.

_____

_____

_____ 2. Assesses the delivery of nursing care in the Emergency Department and identifies problems and any need for improvement.

_____

_____

_____ 3. Assesses the health status of all patients upon arrival in the Emergency Room as outlined in the Nursing Standards.
   3.1 Assesses the patient's immediate needs and data are prioritized accordingly.

_____

_____

   3.2 Obtains pertinent patient history.

_____

_____

   3.3 Completes a patient assessment that includes:
      a. assessment of alterations or deficits in body systems/responses,
      b. assessment of pain associated with any alterations or deficits,

---

*The evaluator is expected to comment on all items rated "U" or "E."

221

    c. patient's perceptions,

    d. knowledge level pertinent to health care.

———————————————————————————————————

3.4 Collects data from patient, family, significant others, health care providers, and by consultation with appropriate personnel.

———————————————————————————————————

3.5 Collects data by interview, observation, inspection, auscultation, and palpation.

———————————————————————————————————

3.6 Interprets and assesses all data collected from reports and records.

———————————————————————————————————

3.7 Organizes assessment data so that they are accurate, complete, and accessible, and so that they remain confidential.

———————————————————————————————————

3.8 Communicates assessment data in an orderly fashion by recording, updating, and verbalizing pertinent information to health team members and to appropriate agencies.

———————————————————————————————————

———————————————————————————————————

II. *Planning:*

——— 1. Serves on hospital committees and helps to plan policies and procedures as directed by Supervisor.

———————————————————————————————————

——— 2. Plans and develops self-objectives.

———————————————————————————————————

——— 3. Plans ways to solve problems and to make improvements in the Emergency Department.

———————————————————————————————————

_____ 4. Formulates an individualized care plan for all patients seen in Emergency Room.

    4.1 Identifies the patient's present/potential problems from the patient assessment:

      a. Data are based on scientific knowledge,

      b. Patient's health status is determined,

      c. Patient's health status is compared to the norm,

      d. Problems are given priority according to impact upon the patient's health status.

    4.2 Formulates desired outcomes, specific to the patient problems and established norms.

    4.3 Establishes desired outcomes that are mutually agreed upon by the nurse, patient, family and significant others and are:

      a. measurable

      b. consistent with other health care providers' expectations

      c. established to restore patient's optimal functioning capabilities

    4.4 Incorporates home health care into patient's desired outcomes. This includes but is not limited to teaching concerning:

      a. disease process/alteration in health status

      b. desired outcomes from health care

      c. complications and prevention

      d. specific signs and symptoms that dictate notifying the health team

      e. medications

      f. diet

      g. exercise/activity

      h. self-care techniques and materials

      i. available support systems and resources

      j. follow-up care

III. _Implementation:_

_____ 1. Implements activities necessary to meeting self-objectives.

_____ 2. Participates in implementing planned changes and activities to improve the Emergency Department.

_____

_____

_____ 3. Holds self accountable for the delivery of quality nursing care.

_____

_____

_____ 4. Promotes harmonious relationships and favorable attitudes among the health care team.

_____

_____

_____ 5. Is knowledgeable of location, care, and operation of all Emergency Department equipment. This includes but is not limited to: Life Pack, sterile trays, crash cart contents, MAST trousers.

_____

_____

_____ 6. Directs Life Flight procedures.

_____

_____

_____ 7. Assists in keeping department clean and organized and restocks supplies as necessary.

_____

_____

_____ 8. Supports and adheres to administrative and nursing service policies and procedures.

_____

_____

_____ 9. Assists with orientation of new employees.

_____

_____

_____ 10. Acts rapidly, effectively, and manages self, patients, and other employees during any emergency situation.

_____

_____

_____ 11. Responds immediately to any emergency within the hospital.

_____

_____

_____ 12. Attends required inservice education programs.

_____

_____

_____ 13. Formulates nursing prescriptions that delineate actions to be taken.
Prescribed actions:
13.1 Are given priority according to desired outcomes.

_____

13.2 Are specific to the patient's problems and desired outcomes.

_____

13.3 Are based on current scientific knowledge.

_____

13.4 Are based on principles of patient teaching.

_____

13.5 Are based on principles of psychosocial interactions.

_____

13.6 Are based on environmental factors influencing patient's health.

_____

13.7 Include human, material, and community resources and support systems.

_____

13.8 Direct achievement of optimal bio-psycho-social status.

_____

13.9 Include keeping the patient, family, and significant others aware of the total health care plan.

_____

_____

_____ 14. Implements actions delineated in the nursing prescriptions. Actions
           implemented:
           14.1 Actively involve the patient, family, and significant others.

           _____

           _____

           14.2 Are consistent with the nursing prescriptions.

           _____

           _____

           14.3 Are based upon current scientific knowledge.

           _____

           _____

           14.4 Are flexible and individualized for each patient.

           _____

           _____

           14.5 Include principles of safety.

           _____

           _____

           14.7 Provide for patient privacy and dignity.

           _____

           _____

           14.8 Reflect a "Patient's Bill of Rights."

           _____

           _____

_____ 15. Conforms to hospital dress code.

           _____

           _____

_____ 16. Is rarely sick or absent from work due to health.

           _____

           _____

_____ 17. Is prompt and attends report.

           _____

           _____

IV. *Evaluation:*

_____ 1. Evaluates self-objectives, revises and formulates new objectives.

_____

_____

_____ 2. Evaluates the effectiveness of problem-solving techniques and activities implemented to improve the Emergency Department.

_____

_____

_____ 3. Contributes to the performance evaluation of nursing personnel in the Emergency Department.

_____

_____

_____ 4. Participates in the evaluation of inservice education offerings.

_____

_____

_____ 5. Evaluates achievement or lack of achievement of desired outcomes.
   5.1 Data are collected concerning the patient's health status.

_____

_____

   5.2 Data are compared to the specific desired outcomes.

_____

_____

   5.3 Includes the patient's evaluation of the achievement of desired outcomes.

_____

_____

_____ 6. From evaluation of achievement or lack of achievement of desired outcomes, reassesses and revises the nursing care plan.
   From evaluation:
   6.1　Reassesses the patient problems.

_____

_____

   6.2　Reassesses desired outcomes to determine if appropriate, realistic, and in correct priority.

_____

_____

6.3   Reassesses nursing prescriptions to determine if appropriate, realistic, and accurately stated.

6.4   Reassesses nursing actions for effectiveness in achieving desired outcomes.

From reassessment:

6.5   Determines new patient present/potential problems.

6.6   From new patient problems, formulates and revises desired outcomes.

6.7   Revises nursing prescriptions.

6.8   Implements new actions in order to carry out revised prescriptions.

6.9   Continually evaluates desired outcomes for achievement or lack of achievement.

6.10 Continually evaluates and revises the nursing care plan according to changes in the patient's health status.

EMERGENCY REGISTERED NURSE: SCORING PROCEDURE

Instructions: Total the number of each item and multiply times the appropriate number. Add these totals to make the score.

$$U \underline{\hspace{2cm}} \times 0 = \underline{\hspace{2cm}}$$

$$S \underline{\hspace{2cm}} \times 1 = \underline{\hspace{2cm}}$$

$$A \underline{\hspace{2cm}} \times 2 = \underline{\hspace{2cm}}$$

$$E \underline{\hspace{2cm}} \times 3 = \underline{\hspace{2cm}} \quad \underline{\hspace{2cm}} \text{ Total Score}$$

Compare total score to the following scale to determine rank:

U	S	A	E
0 to 26	27 to 47	48 to 71	72 to 90

Overall Performance Review Score _____.

ALL ITEMS IN THE FOLLOWING SECTION MUST BE COMPLETED:

A. Interviewer's comments on overall review _____

_____

_____

B. Additional suggestions for overall work improvement and goals for next evaluation _____

_____

_____

C. Self-objectives _____

_____

_____

_____

Date _____ Employee's signature _____

Date _____ Interviewer's signature _____

Date _____ Director of Nursing

EMERGENCY LICENSED PRACTICAL NURSE: JOB DESCRIPTION

Position Requirements:	Graduate from an accredited school for Licensed Practical Nurses with current licensure in the State of Alabama. At least 1 year clinical experience preferred. Membership in the LPN Association desired but not required. Participates in educational conferences and updates and maintains professional knowledge and skills related to the areas of practice.
Position Accountable for:	All nursing care behaviors described in the Emergency Department-Licensed Practical Nurse job description.
Position Accountable to:	Charge Nurse, Supervisor, Director of Nursing Service, patient, and family.
Position Summary:	Performs the functions of a licensed practical nurse in assessing, planning, implementing, and evaluating all assigned patient care in collaboration with the Registered Nurse in the department. Is accountable for all patient care she gives during a shift. Is responsible for adhering to all Standards of Emergency Nursing Care, for managing supplies and equipment with the direction of the Registered Nurse; and for promoting teamwork with physicians and personnel of other departments.

I. *Assessment*

1. Assesses nursing care given by self; identifies problems and need for improvement and communicates this to the Registered Nurse.
2. Assesses the health status of all patients assigned to her promptly upon arrival in Emergency Department as outlined in Nursing Standards.
   2.1 Assists in prioritizing the patient's immediate needs.
   2.2 Completes those portions of the pertinent patient history as directed by the Registered Nurse.
   2.3 Collects data from the patient, family and significant others, health care providers, individuals, and/or agencies in the community.
   2.4 Collects data by: interview, observation, inspection, auscultation, palpation, and reports and records.
   2.5 Organizes assessment data so that they are accurate, complete, and accessible, and so that they remain confidential.
   2.6 Communicates assessment data in an orderly fashion by recording, updating, and communicating to the Registered Nurse and revising as appropriate.

II. *Planning*

    1. Assists in planning policies and procedures when requested.

    2. Plans and develops self-objectives with Supervisor in conjunction with performance evaluation.

    3. Suggests ways to solve problems and make improvements in the department.

    4. In collaboration with the Registered Nurse, contributes to the formulation of patient care plans.

        4.1 Identifies patient problems.

        4.2 Formulates desired outcomes.

        4.3 Communicates the above to the Registered Nurse.

        4.4 Participates with the Registered Nurse in incorporating home health care into desired outcomes.

III. *Implementation*

    1. Implements activities necessary to meeting self-objectives.

    2. Cooperates with the Registered Nurse in implementing planned changes and activities to improve nursing care provided in the department.

    3. Promotes harmonious relationships and favorable attitudes among the health care team.

    4. Is knowledgeable of location, care, and operation of all Emergency Department equipment, including but not limited to: Life Pack, sterile trays, crash cart contents, and MAST trousers.

    5. Assists in maintaining a clean and organized department and restocks supplies as necessary.

    6. Supports and adheres to administrative and nursing service policies and procedures.

    7. Assists with orientation of new employees.

    8. Attends required inservice education programs.

    9. Participates with RN in the implementation of patient's care plans.

    10. Documents nursing actions implemented and effectiveness of implementation in the nurses' notes.

    11. Conforms to hospital dress code.

    12. Is rarely sick or absent from work due to health.

    13. Is prompt and attends report.

IV. *Evaluation*

    1. Evaluates the nursing care she gives.

    2. Evaluates self-objectives and determines need for new objectives.

    3. Participates in the evaluation of policies and procedures.

    4. Evaluates the effectiveness of problem-solving techniques and activities implemented.

    5. Evaluates LPN orientation policies and procedures and recommends revisions.

    6. Participates in the evaluation of inservice education offerings.

    7. Participates with the Registered Nurse in the evaluation and revision of patient's care plans.

EMERGENCY LICENSED PRACTICAL NURSE: PERFORMANCE EVALUATION

Name _____ Employment Date _____

Rating Period _____ To _____

Department _____ Job Title _____

Instructions: Using the following rating scale, indicate the quality of performance by placing the appropriate letter on the line to the left of the item.

U* – Unsatisfactory (does not meet job requirements)
S – Satisfactory (meets job requirements)
A – Above average (exceeds job requirements)
E* – Exceptional performance

I. *Assessment:*

_____ 1. Assesses nursing care given by self; identifies problems and need for improvement and communicates this to the Registered Nurse.

_____

_____

_____ 2. Assesses the health status of all patients assigned to her promptly upon arrival in Emergency Department as outlined in Nursing Standards.
2.1 Assists in prioritizing the patient's immediate needs.

_____

_____

2.2 Completes those portions of the pertinent patient history as directed by the Registered Nurse.

_____

_____

2.3 Collects data from the patient, family and significant others, health care providers, individuals, and/or agencies in the community.

_____

_____

---

*The evaluator is expected to comment on all items rated "U" or "E."

2.4 Collects data by: interview, observation, inspection, auscultation, palpation, and reports and records.

_____

_____

2.5 Organizes assessment data so that they are accurate, complete, and accessible, and so that they remain confidential.

_____

_____

2.6 Communicates assessment data in an orderly fashion by recording, updating, and communicating to the Registered Nurse and revising as appropriate.

_____

_____

II. *Planning:*

_____ 1. Assists in planning policies and procedures when requested.

_____

_____

_____ 2. Plans and develops self-objectives with Supervisor in conjunction with performance evaluation.

_____

_____

_____ 3. Suggests ways to solve problems and to make improvements in the department.

_____

_____

_____ 4. In collaboration with the Registered Nurse, contributes to the formulation of patient care plans.
4.1 Identifies patient problems.

_____

_____

4.2 Formulates desired outcomes.

_____

_____

4.3 Communicates the above to the Registered Nurse.

_____

_____

4.4 Participates with the Registered Nurse in incorporating home health care into desired outcomes.

_____

_____

III. *Implementation:*

_____ 1. Implements activities necessary to meeting self-objectives.

_____

_____ 2. Cooperates with the Registered Nurse in implementing planned changes and activities to improve nursing care provided in the department.

_____

_____

_____ 3. Promotes harmonious relationships and favorable attitudes among the health care team.

_____

_____

_____ 4. Is knowledgeable of location, care, and operation of all Emergency Department equipment, including but not limited to: Life Pack, sterile trays, crash cart contents, and MAST trousers.

_____

_____

_____ 5. Assists in maintaining a clean and organized department and re-stocks supplies as necessary.

_____

_____

_____ 6. Supports and adheres to administrative and nursing service policies and procedures.

_____

_____

_____ 7. Assists with orientation of new employees.

_____

_____

_____ 8. Attends required inservice education programs.

_____

_____

_____ 9. Participates with Registered Nurse in the implementation of patient's care plans.

_____

_____

_____ 10. Documents nursing actions implemented and effectiveness of implementation in the nurses' notes.

_____

_____

_____ 11. Conforms to hospital dress code.

_____

_____

_____ 12. Is rarely sick or absent from work due to health.

_____

_____

_____ 13. Is prompt and attends report.

_____

_____

IV. _Evaluation:_

_____ 1. Evaluates the nursing care she gives.

_____

_____

_____ 2. Evaluates self-objectives and determines need for new objectives.

_____

_____

_____ 3. Participates in the evaluation of policies and procedures.

_____

_____

_____ 4. Evaluates the effectiveness of problem-solving techniques and activities implemented.

_____

_____

_____ 5. Evaluates Licensed Practical Nurse orientation policies and procedures and recommends revisions.

_____

_____

_____ 6. Participates in the evaluation of inservice education offerings.

_____

_____

_____ 7. Participates with the Registered Nurse in the evaluation and revision of patients' care plans.

_____

_____

EMERGENCY LICENSED PRACTICAL NURSE: SCORING PROCEDURE

Instructions: Total the number of each item and multiply times the appropriate number. Add these totals to make the score.

U _____ × 0 = _____

S _____ × 1 = _____

A _____ × 2 = _____

E _____ × 3 = _____   _____ Total Score

Compare total score to the following scale to determine rank:

U	S	A	E
0 to 22	23 to 41	42 to 61	62 to 78

Overall Performance Review Score _____.

ALL ITEMS IN THE FOLLOWING SECTION MUST BE COMPLETED:

A. Interviewer's comments on overall review _____
_____
_____

B. Additional suggestions for overall work improvement and goals for next evaluation _____
_____
_____

C. Self-objectives _____
_____
_____
_____

_____   _____
Date   Employee's signature

_____   _____
Date   Interviewer's signature

_____   _____
Date   Director of Nursing

11

Maternal and Child Health Nursing Practice

STANDARDS OF MATERNAL AND CHILD HEALTH NURSING PRACTICE

Standard I

Data are assessed and gathered concerning the health status of the patient and family throughout the stages of labor, delivery, and postpartum period. This process is complete, continuous, and systematic as evidenced by:

1. *A comprehensive patient history and physical:*

PATIENT INTERVIEW
Reason for admission
a. onset of labor
b. expected delivery date
c. membranes (if ruptured, obtain date, time, color and consistency)
d. plans for anesthesia
e. time and character of contractions
Prenatal data
Allergies
Medications
Past medical history
Cultural, environmental and socioeconomic conditions
Activities of daily living
Personal habits
Last oral intake (fluid and solid)
Food and fluid preferences
Weight gain during pregnancy
Available and accessible human, community, and material resources
Plans for hospitalization (i.e., rooming in, breast feeding, etc.)

PHYSICAL ASSESSMENT
Stage of labor
Cervical
a. Dilatation
b. Effacement
Membranes
a. intact
b. ruptured
Vaginal bleeding
a. normal show
b. bleeding (description)
Contractions
a. frequency
b. duration
c. quality

240

Fetal evaluation
a. fetal heart rate
b. station
c. estimated weeks gestation
d. presentation
e. position

MENTAL STATUS

NUTRITIONAL ASSESSMENT

PERSONAL HYGIENE AND GROOMING

ASSESSMENT DURING DELIVERY
a. physical status
b. mental status

ASSESSMENT DURING POSTPARTUM: PATIENT (MOTHER)
Physical status
Lochia
a. color
b. amount
Pain
a. character
b. relief measures
Mobility
Breasts
a. engorgement
b. nipples
Suture line (episiotomy or cesarian section)

PHYSICAL ASSESSMENT OF NEWBORN IMMEDIATELY FOLLOW-
ING DELIVERY
Apgar at one minute
Apgar at five minutes
Maturity (gestational age)
Placental abnormalities
Congenital abnormalities
Physical assessment of newborn daily (until discharge):
Physical status
a. Respiratory
b. Cardiac
c. Neurological
d. Musculo/skeletal
e. Gastrointestinal
f. GU
g. Skin

*PERCEPTION OF STAGES OF LABOR, DELIVERY, AND
POSTPARTUM PERIOD*
Understanding of labor, delivery, and postpartum period

Desired outcome from hospitalization
Knowledge of care of the newborn
Knowledge of self-care following hospitalization

2. *The collection of data from available sources:*
Patient, family, significant other
Health care providers
Individuals and/or agencies in the community

3. *The collection of data by scientific methodology:*
Interview
Observation
Inspection
Examination
Auscultation
Palpation
Reports and records

4. *The organization of data in a systematic arrangement:*
The arrangement provides:
Accurate collection
Complete collection
Accessibility
Confidentiality

5. *The communication of data in an orderly fashion:*
Data are recorded by each shift, daily.
Data are updated by each shift, daily.
Data are revised and recorded as appropriate.
Data are communicated verbally among health team, daily.

STANDARD II

Nursing care planning consists of determining patient and family's needs and desired outcomes, and preparing the patient for home care. This is evidenced by:

1. *The identification of present/potential patient and family needs, from the assessment:*
Data are grouped into meaningful arrangements, based upon scientific knowledge.
Patient's health status is determined.
Health status is compared to the norms.
Present and potential needs are identified.
Needs are given priority according to impact upon the patient's health status.

2. *The formulation of desired outcomes:*
Patient (family, significant other) and nurse mutually agree upon the patient's and newborn's present/potential health needs.
Patient and nurse mutually agree upon desired outcomes.
Desired outcomes are congruent with the patient and newborn's needs and established norms.
Desired outcomes are specific.

Desired outcomes are measureable within a certain time frame.

Desired outcomes are consistent with other health providers' expectations.

Desired outcomes are established to restore the patient's and family's optimal functioning capabilities.

3. *The incorporation of home health care into the desired outcomes involves teaching concerning:*

Medications

Diet

Exercise/Activity

Self-care techniques and materials

Care of the newborn and materials

Available support systems and resources

STANDARD III

The plan of care is implemented in order to achieve the desired outcome, as evidenced by:

1. *The formulation of nursing prescriptions that delineate actions to be taken. Prescribed actions:*

Are specific to identified patient and family's needs and expected outcomes.

Are based on current scientific knowledge.

Incorporate principles of patient and family teaching.

Incorporate principles of psychosocial interactions.

Incorporate environmental factors influencing the patient's and family's health.

Include human, material, and community resources.

Include keeping patient/family knowledgeable of health status and total health care plan.

2. *The implementation of actions delineated in the nursing prescriptions. Actions implemented:*

Actively involve the patient and family.

Are consistent with the nursing prescriptions.

Are based upon current scientific knowledge.

Are flexible and individualized for each patient and family.

Include principles of safety.

Include principles of infection control.

STANDARD IV

Outcomes of nursing actions are evaluated for further assessment and planning. This is evidenced by:

1. *Evaluating the achievement of desired outcomes:*

Data are collected concerning the patient and newborn's health status.

Data are compared to the specified desired outcomes.

The patient and nurse evaluate the achievement of desired outcomes.

2. *Reassessment of the nursing care plan:*

Outcome of nursing actions directs the reassessment of identified patient and newborn's needs.

Outcome of nursing actions direct reassessment of desired outcomes (assess the desired outcome to determine if appropriate, realistic, and in correct priority).

Outcome of nursing actions direct reassessment of nursing prescriptions (assess the nursing prescriptions to determine if appropriate, realistic, and stated accurately).

Nursing actions are assessed for effectiveness in achieving desired outcomes.

3. *Further planning as directed by the reassessment:*

Reassessment determines new patient and newborn present/potential needs.

New patient and newborn needs direct the formulation and revision of desired outcomes.

Revised desired outcomes direct the revision of nursing prescriptions.

Revised prescriptions direct new actions to be implemented toward desired outcomes.

Desired outcomes are continually evaluated for achievement.

The plan of care is continually evaluated and revised according to changes in the patient/newborn's health status.

MATERNAL AND CHILD HEALTH SUPERVISOR: JOB DESCRIPTION

Position Requirements:	Graduate from an accredited school of nursing with current licensure as a Registered Nurse in the State of Alabama. Two years recent clinical experience in Maternal and Child Health Care. One year supervisory experience.
Professional Requirements:	Pursues programs of continuing education consistent with requirements of the Alabama Nurses' Association. Participates in educational conferences and updates and maintains professional knowledge and skills related to areas of responsibilities.
Position Accountable For:	All nursing care behaviors described in the Maternal and Child Health Supervisor job description.
Position Accountable To:	Director of Nursing, the patient, and family.
Position Summary:	Directs patient care functions and ensures that nursing care is assessed, planned, implemented, and evaluated. Is accountable on a 24-hour basis. Is responsible for meeting the Joint Commission Standards of Patient Care and the established Standards of Maternal and Child Health Nursing Practice, for managing all personnel, supplies, and equipment in the department, and for promoting teamwork with physicians and personnel of the other departments.

I. *Assessment*

1. Assesses the number and level of personnel needed to provide quality patient care in the department and collaborates with the Director of Nursing in adjusting staffing and assignments.
2. Assesses the delivery of nursing care and identifies problems and any needs for improvement.
3. Makes nursing rounds and assesses overall operations of the unit.
4. Ensures that health status of each patient and family is assessed as outlined in the Standards of Maternal and Child Health Nursing Practice Ensures that:
   4.1 A comprehensive patient history and physical is completed, including patient interview, psychological and physical assessment, as well as patient's and family's perception of the stages of labor, delivery, and postpartum period.
   4.2 Data are collected from the patient, family and significant others,

health care providers, and individuals and/or agencies in the community.

   4.3 Data are collected by: interview, observation, inspection, examination, auscultation, palpation, and by reports and records.

   4.4 Assessment data are organized so that they are accurate, complete, and accessible, and so that they remain confidential.

   4.5 Assessment data are communicated in an orderly fashion by reporting, updating, and communicating among the health team daily, and making revisions as appropriate.

II. *Planning*

1. Develops, reviews, and revises all policies and procedures for the Maternal and Child Health Department with approval of the Director of Nursing.

2. Plans and develops self-objectives.

3. Plans ways to solve problems and make improvements in the delivery of patient care.

4. Ensures that each patient and family has a nursing care plan. Plans the care for each patient and family as well as directs and supervises others in the planning of this care. Ensures that:

   4.1 The patient's present/potential needs are identified from the assessment.

   a. Data are based upon current scientific knowledge,

   b. Patient's health status is determined,

   c. Patient's health status is compared to the norm,

   d. Needs are given priority according to the impact on the patient's health status.

   4.2 Desired outcomes are formulated specific to the patient and family problems and established norms.

   4.3 Established desired outcomes are mutually agreed upon by the patient, family, and nurse and are:

   a. Specific

   b. Measurable within a certain time frame

   c. Consistent with other health provider's expectations

   4.4 Home health care is incorporated into the patient's and family's desired outcomes. This includes but is not limited to teaching about the medications, diet, exercise/activity, self-care techniques and materials, care of the newborn, and materials and available support systems and resources.

III. *Implementation*

1. Implements activities necessary to meeting self-objectives.

2. From assessment and identification of problems and needs, implements planned changes and activities to improve the department in collaboration with the Director of Nursing.

3. Promotes the achievement of Maternal and Child Health Department objectives.

4. Ensures that Standards of Maternal and Child Health Nursing Practice are implemented and monitors standards as necessary.

5. Holds self and staff accountable for the delivery of quality nursing care.

6. Acts rapidly and effectively while following hospital policies and procedures and utilizes principles of management during any emergency situation.

7. Promotes harmonious relationships and favorable attitudes among the health care team.

8. Interprets, supports, and recommends administrative and nursing service policies and procedures for employees and ensures compliance. Applies knowledge and skills of management.

9. Assists with orientation of new employees.

10. Keeps the Director of Nursing informed on reportable situations and department needs.

11. Attends required inservice education programs.

12. Implements and directs personnel in implementing the patient's plan of care.

13. Ensures that nursing prescriptions are formulated that delineate actions to be taken. Ensures that prescribed actions:
    13.1 Are specific to the patient's and family's needs and to the desired outcomes.
    13.2 Are based on current scientific knowledge.
    13.3 Incorporate principles of patient and family teaching.
    13.4 Incorporate principles of psychosocial interactions.
    13.5 Incorporate environmental factors influencing the patient's and family's health.
    13.6 Include human, material, and community resources.
    13.7 Include keeping patient and family knowledgeable of health status and total health care plan.

14. Ensures that the actions implemented are delineated in the nursing prescriptions. Actions implemented:
    14.1 Actively involve the patient and family.
    14.2 Are based upon current scientific knowledge.
    14.3 Are flexible and individualized for each patient and family.
    14.4 Include principles of safety.
    14.5 Include principles of infection control.

15. Serves as consultant in technical and professional matters for personnel.

16. Participates and contributes to a unified Quality Assurance Program.

17. Participates in the provision of inservice education programs related to Maternal and Child Health Nursing.

18. Conforms to hospital dress code.

19. Is rarely sick or absent from work due to health.

20. Is prompt and attends report.

21. Serves on hospital committees as requested.

IV. *Evaluation*

1. Continually evaluates the Standards of Maternal and Child Health Nursing Practice by reviewing nursing care plans, assessing patients, reviewing charts, interviewing and observing, participating in Quality Assurance activities and by employing other means of evaluation. Revises standards as appropriate in collaboration with Director of Nursing.

2. Evaluates policies and procedures and revises as necessary.

3. Evaluates self-objectives and determines need for revision and new objectives.

4. Evaluates activities to improve operation of the department and evaluates the effectiveness of problem-solving techniques and approaches.

5. Evaluates the performance of nursing service personnel in the department.

6. Evaluates the achievement of Maternal and Child Health Department objectives in collaboration with Director of Nursing Service.

7. Evaluates orientation policies and procedures and recommends revisions.

8. Evaluates emergencies and any hospital disaster and recommends revisions in policies and procedures and/or need for improvement in employee performance.

9. Evaluates inservice education programs.

10. Ensures that desired outcomes are evaluated for achievement or lack of achievement.

    10.1 Data are collected concerning the patient's health status.

    10.2 Data are compared to the specific desired outcomes.

    10.3 The patient and nurse evaluate the achievement of desired outcomes.

11. Ensures that the nursing care plan is reassessed and revised from the evaluation of achievement or lack of achievement of desired outcomes.

    11.1 Reassesses the patient's needs.

    11.2 Reassesses desired outcomes to determine if appropriate, realistic, and in correct priority.

    11.3 Reassesses nursing prescriptions to determine if appropriate, realistic, and stated accurately.

    11.4 Reassesses nursing actions for effectiveness in achieving desired outcomes.

    From reassessment:

    11.5 Determines new patient present/potential needs.

    11.6 From new patient needs, formulates and revises desired outcomes.

    11.7 Revises nursing prescriptions.

    11.8 Implements new actions in order to carry out revised prescriptions.

    11.9 Continually evaluates nursing actions and desired outcomes for achievement or lack of achievement.

    11.10 Continually evaluates and revises the nursing care plan according to changes in the patient's health status.

MATERNAL AND CHILD HEALTH SUPERVISOR: PERFORMANCE EVALUATION

Name _____ Employment Date _____

Rating Period _____ To _____

Department _____ Job Title _____

Instructions: Using the following rating scale, indicate the quality of performance by placing the appropriate letter on the line to the left of the item.

U* – Unsatisfactory (does not meet job requirements)
S – Satisfactory (meets job requirements)
A – Above average (exceeds job requirements)
E* – Exceptional performance

I. *Assessment:*

_____ 1. Assesses the number and level of personnel needed to provide quality patient care in the department and collaborates with the Director of Nursing in adjusting staffing and assignments.

_____

_____

_____ 2. Assesses the delivery of nursing care and identifies problems and any needs for improvement.

_____

_____

_____ 3. Makes nursing rounds and assesses overall operations of the unit.

_____

_____

_____ 4. Ensures that health status of each patient and family is assessed as outlined in the Standards of Maternal and Child Health Nursing Practice. Ensures that:
   4.1 A comprehensive patient history and physical is completed, including patient interview, psychological and physical assessment, as well as patient's and family's perception of the stages of labor, delivery, and postpartum period.

_____

_____

---

*The evaluator is expected to comment on all items rated "U" or "E."

4.2 Data are collected from the patient, family and significant others, health care providers, and individuals and/or agencies in the community.

_____

_____

4.3 Data are collected by: interview, observation, inspection, examination, auscultation, palpation, and by reports and records.

_____

_____

4.4 Assessment data are organized so that they are accurate, complete, and accessible, and so that they remain confidential.

_____

_____

4.5 Assessment data are communicated in an orderly fashion by reporting, updating, and communicating among the health team daily, and by making revisions as appropriate.

_____

_____

II. _Planning:_

_____ 1. Develops, reviews, and revises all policies and procedures for the Maternal and Child Health Department with approval of the Director of Nursing.

_____

_____

_____ 2. Plans and develops self-objectives.

_____

_____

_____ 3. Plans ways to solve problems and to make improvements in the delivery of patient care.

_____

_____

_____ 4. Ensures that each patient and family has a nursing care plan. Plans the care for each patient and family as well as directs and supervises others in the planning of this care.

Ensures that:

4.1 The patient's present/potential needs are identified from the assessment.

a. Data are based upon current scientific knowledge,

      b. Patient's health status is determined,

      c. Patient's health status is compared to the norm,

      d. Needs are given priority according to the impact on the patient's health status.

_____

_____

4.2 Desired outcomes are formulated specific to the patient and family problems and established norms.

_____

_____

4.3 Established desired outcomes are mutually agreed upon by the patient, family, and nurse and are:

    a. Specific

    b. Measurable within a certain time frame

    c. Consistent with other health providers' expectations

_____

_____

4.4 Home health care is incorporated into the patient's and family's desired outcomes. This includes but is not limited to teaching about the medications, diet, exercise/activity, self-care techniques and materials, care of the newborn, and materials and available support systems and resources.

_____

_____

III. *Implementation:*

_____ 1. Implements activities necessary to meeting self-objectives.

_____

_____

_____ 2. From assessments and identification of problems and needs, implements planned changes and activities to improve the department in collaboration with the Director of Nursing.

_____

_____

_____ 3. Promotes the achievement of Maternal and Child Health Department objectives.

_____

_____

_____ 4. Ensures that Standards of Maternal and Child Health Nursing Practice are implemented and monitors standards as necessary.

_____

_____

_____ 5. Holds self and staff accountable for the delivery of quality nursing care.

_____

_____

_____ 6. Acts rapidly and effectively while following hospital policies and procedures and utilizes principles of management during any emergency situation.

_____

_____

_____ 7. Promotes harmonious relationships and favorable attitudes among the health care team.

_____

_____

_____ 8. Interprets, supports, and recommends administrative and nursing service policies and procedures for employees and ensures compliance. Applies knowledge and skills of management.

_____

_____

_____ 9. Assists with orientation of new employees.

_____

_____

_____ 10 Keeps the Director of Nursing informed on reportable situations and department needs.

_____

_____

_____ 11. Attends required inservice education programs.

_____

_____

_____ 12. Implements and directs personnel in implementing the patient's plan of care.

_____

_____

_____ 13. Ensures that nursing prescriptions are formulated that delineate actions to be taken. Ensures that prescribed actions:

13.1 Are specific to the patient's and family's needs, and to the desired outcomes.

_____

_____

13.2 Are based on current scientific knowledge.

_____

_____

13.3 Incorporate principles of patient and family teaching.

_____

_____

13.4 Incorporate principles of psychosocial interactions.

_____

_____

13.5 Incorporate environmental factors influencing the patient's and family's health.

_____

_____

13.6 Include human, material, and community resources.

_____

_____

13.7 Include keeping patient and family knowledgeable of health status and total health care plan.

_____

_____

_____ 14. Ensures that the actions implemented are delineated in the nursing prescriptions. Actions implemented:

14.1 Actively involve the patient and family.

_____

_____

14.2 Are based upon current scientific knowledge.

_____

_____

14.3 Are flexible and individualized for each patient and family.

_____

_____

14.4 Include principles of safety.

_____

_____

14.5 Include principles of infection control.

_____

_____

_____ 15. Serves as consultant in technical and professional matters for personnel.

_____

_____

_____ 16. Participates and contributes to a unified Quality Assurance Program.

_____

_____

_____ 17. Participates in the provision of inservice education programs related to Maternal and Child Health Nursing.

_____

_____

_____ 18. Conforms to hospital dress code.

_____

_____

_____ 19. Is rarely sick or absent from work due to health.

_____

_____

_____ 20. Is prompt and attends report.

_____

_____

_____ 21. Serves on hospital committees as requested.

_____

_____

IV. _Evaluation:_

_____ 1. Continually evaluates the Standards of Maternal and Child Health Nursing Practice by reviewing nursing care plans, assessing patients, reviewing charts, interviewing and observing, participating in Quality Assurance activities, and by employing other means of evaluation. Revises standards as appropriate in collaboration with Director of Nursing.

———————————————————————————

———— 2. Evaluates policies and procedures and revises as necessary.

———————————————————————————

———— 3. Evaluates self-objectives and determines need for revision and new objectives.

———————————————————————————

———— 4. Evaluates activities to improve operation of the department and evaluates the effectiveness of problem-solving techniques and approaches.

———————————————————————————

———— 5. Evaluates the performance of nursing service personnel in the department.

———————————————————————————

———— 6. Evaluates the achievement of Maternal and Child Health Department objectives in collaboration with Director of Nursing Service.

———————————————————————————

———— 7. Evaluates orientation policies and procedures and recommends revisions.

———————————————————————————

———— 8. Evaluates emergencies and any hospital disaster and recommends revisions in policies and procedures and/or need for improvement in employee performance.

———————————————————————————

———— 9. Evaluates inservice education programs.

———————————————————————————

_____ 10. Ensures that desired outcomes are evaluated for achievement or lack of achievement.

10.1 Data are collected concerning the patient's health status.

_____

_____

10.2 Data are compared to the specific desired outcomes.

_____

_____

10.3 The patient and nurse evaluate the achievement of desired outcomes.

_____

_____

_____ 11. Ensures that the nursing care plan is reassessed and revised from the evaluation of achievement or lack of achievement of desired outcomes.
From evaluation:
11.1   Reassesses the patient's needs.

_____

_____

11.2   Reassesses desired outcomes to determine if appropriate, realistic, and in correct priority.

_____

_____

11.3   Reassesses nursing prescriptions to determine if appropriate, realistic, and stated accurately.

_____

_____

11.4   Reassesses nursing actions for effectiveness in achieving desired outcomes.

_____

_____

From reassessment:
11.5   Determines new patient present/potential needs.

_____

_____

11.6   From new patient needs, formulates and revises desired outcomes.

_____

_____

11.7   Revises nursing prescriptions.

11.8   Implements new actions in order to carry out revised pre-
        scriptions.

11.9   Continually evaluates nursing actions and desired outcomes
        for achievement or lack of achievement.

11.10   Continually evaluates and revises the nursing care plan ac-
        cording to changes in the patient's health status.

MATERNAL AND CHILD HEALTH SUPERVISOR: SCORING PROCEDURE

Instructions: Total the number of each item and multiply times the appropriate number. Add these totals to make the score.

U _____×0=_____

S _____×1=_____

A _____×2=_____

E _____×3=_____   _____ Total Score

Compare total score to the following scale to determine rank:

U	S	A	E
0 to 34	35 to 61	62 to 93	94 to 117

Overall Performance Review Score _____.

ALL ITEMS IN THE FOLLOWING SECTION MUST BE COMPLETED:

A. Interviewer's comments on overall review _____

_____

_____

B. Additional suggestions for overall work improvement and goals for next evaluation _____

_____

_____

C. Self-objectives _____

_____

_____

_____

_____ Date   Employee's signature

_____ Date   Interviewer's signature

_____ Date   Director of Nursing

MATERNAL AND CHILD HEALTH REGISTERED NURSE: JOB DESCRIPTION

Position Requirements:	Graduate from an accredited school of nursing with current licensure as a registered nurse in the State of Alabama. Specific orientation for Maternal and Child Health Care.
Professional Requirements:	Pursues programs of continuing education consistent with requirements of the Alabama Nurses' Association. Participates in educational conferences and updates and maintains professional knowledge and skills related to areas of responsibilities.
Position Accountable for:	All nursing care behaviors described in the Maternal and Child Health registered nurse job description.
Position Accountable to:	Supervisor, Director of Nursing, the patient, and family.
Position Summary:	Performs the primary functions of a registered nurse in assessing, planning, implementing, and evaluating the care of patients in the department (prepartum, labor, delivery, postpartum, and nursery) during her shift. Is responsible for meeting the established Standards of Maternal and Child Health Nursing Practice, for managing all assigned personnel, supplies, and equipment in the department, and for promoting team work with physicians and personnel of other departments.

I. *Assessment*

1. Assesses the number and level of personnel needed to provide quality patient care in the department and collaborates with the Supervisor in adjusting staffing and assignments.
2. Assesses the delivery of nursing care in the department and identifies problems and any need for improvement.
3. Assesses the health status of each patient and family as outlined in the Standards of Maternal and Child Health Nursing Practice.
   3.1 Completes a comprehensive patient history and physical including patient interview, psychological and physical assessment, as well as patient's and family's perception of the stages of labor, delivery, and postpartum period.
   3.2 Collects data from the patient, family and significant others, health care providers, and individuals and/or agencies in the community.

3.3 Collects data by: interview, observation, inspection, examination, auscultation, palpation, and by reports and records.

3.4 Organizes assessment data so that they are accurate, complete, and accessible, and so that they remain confidential.

3.5 Communicates assessment data in an orderly fashion by reporting, updating, and communicating among the health team daily, and by revising as appropriate.

II. *Planning*

1. Serves on hospital committees and helps to plan policies and procedures, as directed by the Supervisor.

2. Plans and develops self-objectives.

3. Plans ways to solve problems and to make improvements on the unit, in collaboration with the Supervisor.

4. Completes a written nursing care plan for each patient and family. Plans the care for each patient and family as well as directs and supervises others in the planning of this care.

   4.1 Identifies the patient's and family's present/potential needs from the assessment.

   4.2 Formulates desired outcomes, specific to the patient and family problems and established norms.

   4.3 Ensures that desired outcomes are mutually agreed upon by the patient, family, and nurse and are specific, measureable within a certain time frame, and consistent with other health providers' expectations.

   4.4 Incorporates home health care into patient's and family's desired outcomes. This includes but is not limited to teaching about the medications, diet, exercise/activity, self-care techniques and materials, care of the newborn, and materials and available support systems and resources.

III. *Implementation*

1. Implements activities necessary to meeting self-objectives.

2. Participates in implementing planned change and activities to improve the department.

3. Participates in activities promoting the achievement of Maternal and Child Health Department objectives.

4. Holds self and staff accountable for the delivery of quality nursing care.

5. Acts rapidly and effectively and manages self, patients, and other employees during any emergency situation.

6. Supports and adheres to administrative and nursing service policies and procedures.

7. Promotes harmonious relationships and favorable attitudes among the health care team.

8. Assists with orientation of new employees.

9. Is knowledgeable of Maternal and Child Department equipment. This includes but is not limited to: fetal heart monitor, sterile trays, adult

and newborn crash cart contents, incubator, isolette, and Ohio warmer.

10. Attends required inservice education programs.
11. Formulates nursing prescriptions that delineate actions to be taken. Prescribed Actions:
    11.1 Are specific to the patient's and family's needs, and to the desired outcomes.
    11.2 Are based on scientific knowledge.
    11.3 Are based on current principles of patient and family teaching.
    11.4 Are based on current principles of psychosocial interactions.
    11.5 Are based on environmental factors influencing the patient's and family's health.
    11.6 Include human, material, and community resources.
    11.7 Include keeping patient and family knowledgeable of health status and total health care plan.
12. Implements the actions delineated in the nursing prescriptions. Actions implemented:
    12.1 Actively involve the patient and family.
    12.2 Are based on current scientific knowledge.
    12.3 Are flexible and individualized for each patient and family.
    12.4 Include principles of safety.
    12.5 Include principles of infection control.
13. Conforms to hospital dress code.
14. Is rarely sick or absent from work due to health.
15. Is prompt and attends report.

IV. *Evaluation*
1. Evaluates self-objectives, revises and formulates new objectives.
2. Evaluates the effectiveness of problem-solving techniques and activities implemented to improve the department.
3. Contributes to the performance evaluation of nursing service personnel in the department.
4. Participates in the evaluation of inservice education programs.
5. Evaluates achievement or lack of achievement of desired outcomes.
    5.1 Data are collected concerning the patient's health status.
    5.2 Data are compared to the specific desired outcomes.
    5.3 The nurse and patient evaluate the achievement of desired outcomes.
6. From evaluation of achievement or lack of achievement of desired outcomes, reassesses and revises the nursing care plan.
    From evaluation:
    6.1 Reassesses the patient needs.
    6.2 Reassesses desired outcomes to determine if appropriate, realistic, and in correct priority.
    6.3 Reassesses nursing prescriptions to determine if appropriate, realistic, and stated accurately.
    6.4 Reassesses nursing actions for effectiveness in achieving desired outcomes.

From reassessment:

6.5   Determines new patient present/potential needs.

6.6   From new patient needs, formulates and revises desired out-
      comes.

6.7   Revises nursing prescriptions.

6.8   Implements new actions in order to carry out revised prescrip-
      tions.

6.9   Continually evaluates desired outcomes for achievement or lack
      of achievement.

6.10 Continually evaluates and revises the nursing care plan according
      to changes in the patient's health status.

MATERNAL AND CHILD HEALTH REGISTERED NURSE: PERFORMANCE EVALUATION

Name _____ Employment Date _____

Rating Period _____ To _____

Department _____ Job Title _____

Instructions: Using the following rating scale, indicate the quality of performance by placing the appropriate letter on the line to the left of the item.

U* – Unsatisfactory (does not meet job requirements)
S – Satisfactory (meets job requirements)
A – Above average (exceeds job requirements)
E* – Exceptional performance

I. *Assessment:*

_____ 1. Assesses the number and level of personnel needed to provide quality patient care in the department and collaborates with the Supervisor in adjusting staffing and assignments.

_____

_____

_____ 2. Assesses the delivery of nursing care in the department and identifies problems and any need for improvement.

_____

_____

_____ 3. Assesses the health status of each patient and family as outlined in the Standards of Maternal and Child Health Nursing Practice.
    3.1 Completes comprehensive patient history and physical, including patient interview, psychological and physical assessment, as well as patient's and family's perception of the stages of labor, delivery, and postpartum period.

_____

_____

    3.2 Collects data from the patient, family and significant others, health care providers, and individuals and/or agencies in the community.

_____

_____

---

*The evaluator is expected to comment on all items rated "U" or "E."

3.3 Collects data by: interview, observation, inspection, examination, auscultation, palpation, and by reports and records.

_____

3.4 Organizes assessment data so that they are accurate, complete, and accessible, and so that they remain confidential.

_____

3.5 Communicates assessment data in an orderly fashion by reporting, updating, and communicating among the health team daily, and by revising as appropriate.

_____

_____

II. *Planning:*

_____ 1. Serves on hospital committees and helps to plan policies and procedures as directed by the Supervisor.

_____

_____ 2. Plans and develops self-objectives.

_____

_____ 3. Plans ways to solve problems and to make improvements on the unit, in collaboration with the Supervisor.

_____

_____ 4. Completes a written nursing care plan for each patient and family. Plans the care for each patient and family as well as directs and supervises others in the planning of this care.
4.1 Identifies the patient's and family's present/potential needs from the assessment.

_____

4.2 Formulates desired outcomes, specific to the patient and family problems and established norms.

_____

_____

4.3 Ensures that desired outcomes are mutually agreed upon by the patient, family, and nurse and are specific, measurable within a certain time frame, and consistent with other health providers' expectations.

_____

_____

4.4 Incorporates home health care into patient's and family's desired outcomes. This includes but is not limited to teaching about the medications, diet, exercise/activity, self-care techniques and materials, care of the newborn, and materials and available support systems and resources.

_____

_____

III. _Implementation:_

_____ 1. Implements activities necessary to meeting self-objectives.

_____

_____ 2. Participates in implementing planned change and activities to improve the department.

_____

_____ 3. Participates in activities promoting the achievement of Maternal and Child Health Department objectives.

_____

_____ 4. Holds self and staff accountable for the delivery of quality nursing care.

_____

_____ 5. Acts rapidly and effectively and manages self, patients, and other employees during any emergency situation.

_____

_____ 6. Supports and adheres to administrative and nursing service policies and procedures.

_____

_____

_____ 7. Promotes harmonious relationships and favorable attitudes among the health care team.

_____

_____

_____ 8. Assists with orientation of new employees.

_____

_____

_____ 9. Is knowledgeable of Maternal and Child Health Department equipment. This includes but is not limited to: fetal heart monitor, sterile trays, adult and newborn crash cart contents, incubator, isolette, and Ohio warmer.

_____

_____

_____ 10. Attends required inservice education programs.

_____

_____

_____ 11. Formulates nursing prescriptions that delineate actions to be taken. Prescribed actions:
    11.1 Are specific to the patient's and family's needs, and to the desired outcomes.

_____

_____

    11.2 Are based on scientific knowledge.

_____

_____

    11.3 Are based on current principles of patient and family teaching.

_____

_____

    11.4 Are based on current principles of psychosocial interactions.

_____

_____

    11.5 Are based on environmental factors influencing the patient's and family's health.

_____

_____

    11.6 Include human, material, and community resources.

_____

_____

11.7 Include keeping patient and family knowledgeable of health status and total health care plan.

_____

_____

_____ 12. Implements the actions delineated in the nursing prescriptions. Actions implemented:

12.1 Actively involve the patient and family.

_____

12.2 Are based on current scientific knowledge.

_____

12.3 Are flexible and individualized for each patient and family.

_____

12.4 Include principles of safety.

_____

12.5 Include principles of infection control.

_____

_____

_____ 13. Conforms to hospital dress code.

_____

_____

_____ 14. Is rarely sick or absent from work due to health.

_____

_____

_____ 15. Is prompt and attends report.

_____

_____

IV. _Evaluation:_

_____ 1. Evaluates self-objectives, revises and formulates new objectives.

_____

_____

_____ 2. Evaluates the effectiveness of problem-solving techniques and activities implemented to improve the department.

_____

_____

_____ 3. Contributes to the performance evaluation of nursing service personnel in the department.

_____

_____

_____ 4. Participates in the evaluation of inservice education programs.

_____

_____

_____ 5. Evaluates achievement or lack of achievement of desired outcomes.
　　　5.1 Data are collected concerning the patient's health status.

_____

_____

　　　5.2 Data are compared to the specific desired outcomes.

_____

_____

　　　5.3 The nurse and patient evaluate the achievement of desired outcomes.

_____

_____

_____ 6. From evaluation of achievement or lack of achievement of desired outcomes, reassesses and revises the nursing care plan.
　　　From evaluation:
　　　6.1 Reassesses the patient needs.

_____

_____

　　　6.2 Reassesses desired outcomes to determine if appropriate, realistic, and in correct priority.

_____

_____

　　　6.3 Reassesses nursing prescriptions to determine if appropriate, realistic, and stated accurately.

_____

_____

6.4 Reassesses nursing actions for effectiveness in achieving desired outcomes.

_____

_____

From reassessment:
 6.5 Determines new patient present/potential needs.

_____

 6.6 From new patient needs, formulates and revises desired outcomes.

_____

 6.7 Revises nursing prescriptions.

_____

 6.8 Implements new actions in order to carry out revised prescriptions.

_____

 6.9 Continually evaluates desired outcomes for achievement or lack of achievement.

_____

6.10 Continually evaluates and revises the nursing care plan according to changes in the patient's health status.

_____

_____

MATERNAL AND CHILD HEALTH REGISTERED NURSE: SCORING PROCEDURE

Instructions: Total the number of each item and multiply times the appropriate number. Add these totals to make the score.

U _____ ×0=_____

S _____ ×1=_____

A _____ ×2=_____

E _____ ×3=_____   _____ Total Score

Compare total score to the following scale to determine rank:

U	S	A	E
0 to 24	25 to 44	45 to 66	67 to 84

Overall Performance Review Score _____.

ALL ITEMS IN THE FOLLOWING SECTION MUST BE COMPLETED:

A. Interviewer's comments on overall review _____
_____
_____

B. Additional suggestions for overall work improvement and goals for next evaluation _____
_____
_____

C. Self-objectives _____
_____
_____
_____

_____   _____
Date   Employee's signature

_____   _____
Date   Interviewer's signature

_____   _____
Date   Director of Nursing

MATERNAL AND CHILD HEALTH LICENSED PRACTICAL NURSE: JOB DESCRIPTION

Position Requirements:	Graduate from an accredited school of nursing with current licensure as a Licensed Practical Nurse in the State of Alabama. Pursues programs of continuing education. Participates in educational conferences and updates and maintains knowledge and skills related to areas of responsibilities.
Position Accountable for:	All nursing behaviors described in the Maternal and Child Health Licensed Practical Nurse job description.
Position Accountable to:	Supervisor of Maternal and Child Health Department, RN in charge, Director of Nursing, the patient, and family.
Position Summary:	Performs functions of Licensed Practical Nurse in assessing, planning, implementing, and evaluating the care of assigned patients during her shift under the supervision of an RN. Is responsible for adhering to the Standards of Maternal and Child Health Nursing Practice, for managing supplies and equipment on the unit, and for promoting team work with physicians and personnel of other departments.

I. *Assessment*

1. Assesses nursing care given by self; identifies problems and need for improvement and communicates this to the Registered Nurse.
2. Assesses the health status of patients included in her assignment as outlined in the Standards of Maternal Child Health Nursing Practice.
   2.1 Completes those portions of the patient assessment as directed by the Registered Nurse.
   2.2 Collects data from the patient, family and significant other, health care providers, individuals, and/or agencies in the community.
   2.3 Collects data by: interview, observation, inspection, auscultation, palpation, and reports and records.
   2.4 Organizes assessment data so that they are accurate, complete, and accessible, and so that they remain confidential.
   2.5 Communicates assessment data in an orderly fashion by: recording, updating, and communicating among the health team, and by revising data as appropriate.

II. *Planning*

 1. Helps to plan, review and revise policies and procedures as requested.
 2. Plans and develops self-objectives with Supervisor in conjunction with performance evaluation.
 3. Suggests ways to solve problems and to make improvements in the department.
 4. Under the direction of the RN contributes to the formulation of patient and family care plans as outlined in the nursing standards.
    4.1 Identifies patient and family needs.
    4.2 Formulates desired outcomes.
    4.3 Communicates any deviation from the norm to health team members.

III. *Implementation*

 1. Implements activities necessary to meeting self-objectives.
 2. Cooperates with the Supervisor in implementing planned change and activities to improve nursing care in the department.
 3. Promotes harmonious relationships and favorable attitudes among the health care team.
 4. Supports and adheres to administrative and nursing service policies and procedures.
 5. Assists with orientation of new employees.
 6. Is knowledgeable of equipment, manages self, and assists with management of assigned patients during emergencies.
 7. Attends required inservice education programs.
 8. Participates with the Registered Nurse in the implementation of assigned patient's and family's plan of care.
 9. Documents nursing actions implemented and effectiveness of implementation, in the nurses' notes.
10. Conforms to hospital dress code.
11. Is rarely sick or absent from work due to health.
12. Is prompt and attends report.

IV. *Evaluation*

 1. Evaluates the nursing care she gives.
 2. Evaluates self-objectives and determines need for new objectives.
 3. Evaluates the effectiveness of problem-solving techniques and activities implemented to improve nursing care in the department.
 4. Evaluates LPN orientation policies and procedures and recommends revisions.
 5. Participates in the evaluation of inservice education programs.
 6. Participates with the RN in the evaluation and revision of assigned patients' and families' care plans.

MATERNAL AND CHILD HEALTH LICENSED PRACTICAL NURSE: PERFORMANCE EVALUATION

Name _____ Employment Date _____

Rating Period _____ To _____

Department _____ Job Title _____

Instructions: Using the following rating scale, indicate the quality of performance by placing the appropriate letter on the line to the left of the item.

    U* – Unsatisfactory (does not meet job requirements)
    S – Satisfactory (meets job requirements)
    A – Above average (exceeds job requirements)
    E* – Exceptional performance

I. *Assessment:*

_____ 1. Assesses nursing care given by self; identifies problems and need for improvement and communicates this to the Registered Nurse.

_____

_____

_____ 2. Assesses the health status of patients included in her assignment as outlined in the Standards of Maternal and Child Health Nursing Practice.

2.1 Completes those portions of the patient assessment as directed by the Registered Nurse.

_____

_____

2.2 Collects data from the patient, family and significant other, health care providers, individuals, and/or agencies in the community.

_____

_____

2.3 Collects data by: interview, observation, inspection, auscultation, palpation, and reports and records.

_____

_____

---

*The evaluator is expected to comment on all items rated "U" or "E."

2.4 Organizes assessment data so that they are accurate, complete, and accessible, and so that they remain confidential.

_____

_____

2.5 Communicates assessment data in an orderly fashion by: recording, updating, communicating among the health team, and by revising data as appropriate.

_____

_____

II. *Planning:*

_____ 1. Helps to plan, review and revise policies and procedures as requested.

_____

_____

_____ 2. Plans and develops self-objectives with Supervisor in conjunction with performance evaluation.

_____

_____

_____ 3. Suggests ways to solve problems and to make improvements in the department.

_____

_____

_____ 4. Under the direction of the Registered Nurse contributes to the formulation of patient and family care plans as outlined in the Nursing Standards.
4.1 Identifies patient and family needs.

_____

_____

4.2 Formulates desired outcomes.

_____

_____

4.3 Communicates any deviation from the norm to health team members.

_____

_____

III. *Implementation:*

_____ 1. Implements activities necessary to meeting self-objectives.

_____

_____

_____ 2. Cooperates with the Supervisor in implementing planned changes and activities to improve nursing care in the department.

_____

_____

_____ 3. Promotes harmonious relationships and favorable attitudes among the health care team.

_____

_____

_____ 4. Supports and adheres to administrative and nursing service policies and procedures.

_____

_____

_____ 5. Assists with orientation of new employees.

_____

_____

_____ 6. Is knowledgeable of equipment, manages self, and assists with management of assigned patients during emergencies.

_____

_____

_____ 7. Attends required inservice education programs.

_____

_____

_____ 8. Participates with the Registered Nurse in the implementation of assigned patient's and family's plan of care.

_____

_____

_____ 9. Documents nursing actions implemented and effectiveness of implementation in the nurses' notes.

_____

_____

_____ 10. Conforms to hospital dress code.

_____

_____

_____ 11. Is rarely sick or absent from work due to health.

_____

_____

_____ 12. Is prompt and attends report.

_____

_____

IV. *Evaluation:*

_____ 1. Evaluates the nursing care she gives.

_____

_____

_____ 2. Evaluates self-objectives and determines need for new objectives.

_____

_____

_____ 3. Evaluates the effectiveness of problem-solving techniques and activities implemented to improve nursing care in the department.

_____

_____

_____ 4. Evaluates Licensed Practical Nurse orientation policies and procedures and recommends revisions.

_____

_____

_____ 5. Participates in the evaluation of inservice education programs.

_____

_____

_____ 6. Participates with the Registered Nurse in the evaluation and revision of assigned patient's and family's care plans.

_____

_____

MATERNAL AND CHILD HEALTH LICENSED PRACTICAL NURSE: SCORING PROCEDURE

Instructions: Total the number of each item and multiply times the appropriate number. Add these totals to make the score.

U _____ × 0 = _____

S _____ × 1 = _____

A _____ × 2 = _____

E _____ × 3 = _____   _____ Total Score

Compare total score to the following scale to determine rank:

U	S	A	E
0 to 21	22 to 37	38 to 57	58 to 72

Overall Performance Review Score _____.

ALL ITEMS IN THE FOLLOWING SECTION MUST BE COMPLETED:

A. Interviewer's comments on overall review _____
_____
_____

B. Additional suggestions for overall work improvement and goals for next evaluation _____
_____
_____

C. Self-objectives _____
_____
_____
_____

_____   _____
Date   Employee's signature

_____   _____
Date   Interviewer's signature

_____   _____
Date   Director of Nursing

12

Administrative Job Descriptions and Performance Evaluations

DIRECTOR OF NURSING SERVICE: JOB DESCRIPTION

Position Requirements: Graduate of an accredited school of nursing with current licensure as a registered nurse in the State of Alabama. Bachelor of Science Degree required; Master's Degree preferred, with demonstrated ability in nursing practice and administration. Four years recent clinical experience required, including 1 year supervisory experience.

Position Accountable for: All behavior described in the Director of Nursing Service job description.

Position Accountable to: Administrator, patient, and family.

Position Summary: Under the direction of the Administrator, is responsible for management of the nursing service department and for the direction and supervision of all nursing service functions and activities. Is responsible for the quality of patient care and ensures that sufficient and properly prepared personnel carry out the functions of Nursing Service. Is knowledgeable of social, economical, and legal issues effecting the health care systems and seeks all opportunities for keeping staff up to date in health care practices. Develops, directs the implementation, and ensures compliance of Standards of Nursing Practice that promote optimum health care delivery.

PRINCIPLE RESPONSIBILITIES AND DUTIES:

I. *Assessment*
1. Collects and analyzes data to determine staffing patterns and overall Nursing Service staffing plans. Uses these data to project staffing needs, to hire personnel, and to ensure that all nursing units are staffed according to patient needs.
2. Reviews work schedules, assignments, patient classification, and supervisor's reports to assess daily the appropriate number and level of personnel needed to provide quality care. Recommends and carries out changes in personnel and assignments accordingly.
3. Makes nursing rounds to assess the quality of patient care and to identify problems and needs.

4. Investigates complaints concerning nursing service and takes appropriate action.
5. With the Infection Control Nurse, assesses nursing care, the environment, and equipment regularly to ensure high standards of cleanliness, safety, and infection control.

II. *Planning*
   1. Plans and develops self-objectives, identifies areas of delegation, sets priorities and target dates for completion, and identifies resources needed.
   2. Serves as manager, communicator, participator in institutional policy development and planning, and as evaluator of nursing care.
   3. Organizes, plans, and directs department functions and activities to comply with long- and short-term objectives, and with hospital philosophy and policies.
   4. Establishes (with assistance of management personnel) the department philosophy, goals and objectives, standards, and policies and procedures to achieve high quality nursing care.
   5. Coordinates nursing's role and it's relationship to other departments in the hospital, as well as the Medical Staff.
   6. Organizes department structure, interprets this relationship to nursing personnel; plans, directs, and supervises the nursing service.
   7. Develops (with assistance of management personnel) job/position descriptions that are criteria based and have specific performance evaluations that relate to each job description.
   8. Develops policies and procedures regarding qualifications and employment of nursing staff members.
   9. Establishes and maintains an effective patient classification system.
   10. Develops a system for evaluation of work performance and evaluates the performance of management personnel accordingly; sees that this system is maintained and that workers are evaluated in a fair and objective manner.
   11. Plans ways to promote the growth and development of personnel through inservice programs, workshops, seminars, and other continuing education opportunities.
   12. Assists in establishing and maintaining a safety, fire, and disaster program in cooperation with administration and safety committee and assures proper handling and emergency care of patients, personnel, and visitors involved in accidents.
   13. Outlines and interprets to personnel nursing service's role in disaster planning.
   14. Serves on committees including but not limited to: Department Head Meetings, Medical Staff Committee (serves as formal liasion with the Medical Staff), Hospital Quality Assurance Committee, Infection Control, Safety, Pharmacy and Therapeutics, Medical Records, Institutional Planning Meetings, Nursing Education Committee, Nursing Quality Assurance, Nursing Policy and Procedure Committee, and Li-

brary Committee; attends Hospital Board Meetings to represent Nursing Service, attends nursing staff meetings and inservice education meetings.

15. Plans ways to improve leadership skills and to anticipate and minimize problems, and ways to identify these problems and to plan their resolution.

III. *Implementation*

1. Directs the formulation and implementation of policies, procedures, and standards of practice.
2. Conducts monthly management meetings.
3. Meets regularly with the Administrator to discuss objectives, staffing needs, budget, hospital policies, and management problems.
4. Maintains compliance with nursing care standards, hospital policies and procedures, and regulatory agency requirements.
5. Interprets nursing to hospital administration, medical staff, and related public.
6. Interprets policies, procedures, objectives, standards, philosophy, and other matters to personnel.
7. Interviews applicants for nursing positions, approves applicants for hiring, and terminates personnel when necessary.
8. Implements activities necessary to meet nursing objectives, as well as self-objectives.
9. Promotes harmonious relationships and favorable attitudes among the health care team.
10. Serves as consultant and role model for nursing personnel.
11. Initiates planned change and evaluates outcome to ensure that care is safe, efficient, and therapeutic.
12. In collaboration with Inservice Director, orients, instructs, and trains new personnel in nursing functions, policies, and procedures.
13. Assists and supports Inservice Director in conducting regular inservice meetings and in providing continuing education for personnel.
14. Ensures that regular staff meetings are held for all levels of personnel.
15. Establishes a system of record keeping and keeps personnel records current.
16. Maintains direct patient contact and involvement in patient care.
17. Investigates problems, irregularities, and policy violations and takes corrective action and follow-up when necessary.
18. Serves as consultant on hospital admitting and discharge procedures, and other matters that affect patient care (or nursing service).
19. Prepares and submits budget information to administration.
20. Ensures that management personnel provide unit orientation, education, and meetings on a regular basis; evaluate personnel, assess supply and equipment needs, and maintain adequate stock of supplies.

21. Assist management personnel in developing patient care plans and supervising other personnel in this area; in providing for psychosocial and spiritual needs of the patients; in helping unit personnel to maintain good mental, physical, and psychological health; in solving grievances and problems.

22. Assists management personnel in developing objectives, planned change, policy and procedure development, and monitoring of standards of nursing care.

23. Keeps informed and up-to-date in all aspects of nursing care and management through literature, workshops, seminars, courses, and conferences with other nursing directors.

24. Maintains adequate reference library available to nursing personnel.

25. Maintains contact and communication with Administrator, department heads, and Medical Staff concerning all areas of direct and indirect patient care and hospital matters.

26. Conforms to hospital dress code.

27. Is rarely sick or absent from work due to health.

IV. *Evaluation*

1. Evaluates and submits a report monthly concerning the functioning and progress of nursing service. Submits evaluation of achievement of goals and objectives, accomplishments, problems, and unusual happenings to the Administrator.

2. Evaluates and analyzes incident reports and takes the appropriate follow-up action.

3. Continually evaluates the care delivered by regular review of Management Reports, direct observation and patient rounds, results from QA studies, review of charts and care plans, results of monitoring standards, patient questionnaires, and by other sources. Ensures continual corrective and follow-up action where deficient.

4. Evaluates and revises goals and objectives, as well as self-objectives.

5. Evaluates the performance of supervisors and head nurses according to their job descriptions.

6. Evaluates patient classification and staffing on a regular basis and revises as necessary.

7. Evaluates and revises forms to be used in nursing department or that affect nursing service.

8. Evaluates facilities and equipment used in the department.

9. Oversees actions of Nursing Quality Assurance Committee and sees that all pertinent information is related to the hospital-wide QA program.

10. Evaluates and revises policies and procedures.

11. Evaluates the effectiveness of problem-solving techniques.

12. Evaluates personnel's performance during emergencies and hospital disasters.

13. Constantly evaluates attitudes, morale, and interpersonal relationships and promotes ways to improve in these areas.

14. Evaluates effectiveness of orientation and staff development programs.
15. Evaluates and ensures that nursing process is carried out in a continuous manner on all patients.

SUPERVISORY RELATIONSHIPS

Directly supervises:

Inservice Director
Infection Control Nurse
Day Shift Supervisor
Evening Supervisor
Night Supervisor
Head Nurses (relief supervisors)
ICCU Supervisor
OR/RR Supervisor
OB Supervisor
ER Supervisor
Central Service Supervisor
Nursing Service Secretary

Indirectly supervises:

Staff Registered Nurse
Staff Licensed Practical Nurse
ICCU, ER, OB, and OR/RR
personnel
Nursing Assistants
Unit Secretaries
Orderlies
CSR Technicians
Surgical Technicians

DIRECTOR OF NURSING SERVICE: PERFORMANCE EVALUATION

Name _____ Employment Date _____

Rating Period _____ To _____

Department _____ Job Title _____

Instructions: Using the following rating scale, indicate the quality of performance by placing the appropriate letter on the line to the left of the item.

U* – Unsatisfactory (does not meet job requirements)
S – Satisfactory (meets job requirements)
A – Above average (exceeds job requirements)
E* – Exceptional performance

I. *Assessment:*

_____ 1. Collects and analyzes data to determine staffing patterns and overall Nursing Service staffing plans. Uses these data to project staffing needs, to hire personnel, and to ensure that all nursing units are staffed according to patient needs.

_____

_____

_____ 2. Reviews work schedules, assignments, patient classification, and Supervisors' reports to assess daily the appropriate number and level of personnel needed to provide quality care. Recommends and carries out changes in personnel and assignments accordingly.

_____

_____

_____ 3. Makes nursing rounds to assess the quality of patient care and to identify problems and needs.

_____

_____

_____ 4. Investigates complaints concerning Nursing Service and takes appropriate action.

_____

_____

---

*The evaluator is expected to comment on all items rated "U" or "E."

_____ 5. With the Infection Control Nurse, assesses nursing care, the environment, and equipment regularly to ensure high standards of cleanliness, safety, and infection control.

_____

_____

II. _Planning:_

_____ 1. Plans and develops self-objectives, identifies areas of delegation, sets priorities and target dates for completion, and identifies resources needed.

_____

_____

_____ 2. Serves as manager, communicator, participator in institutional policy development and planning, and as evaluator of nursing care.

_____

_____

_____ 3. Organizes, plans, and directs department functions and activities to comply with long- and short-term objectives, and with hospital philosophy and policies.

_____

_____

_____ 4. Establishes (with assistance of management personnel) the department philosophy, goals and objectives, standards, and policies and procedures to achieve high quality nursing care.

_____

_____

_____ 5. Coordinates nursing's role and its relationship to other departments in the hospital as well as with the medical staff.

_____

_____

_____ 6. Organizes department structure, interprets this relationship to nursing personnel; plans, directs, and supervises the Nursing Service.

_____

_____

_____ 7. Develops (with assistance of management personnel) job/position descriptions that are criteria based and have specific performance evaluations that relate to each job description.

_____

_____

_____ 8. Develops policies and procedures regarding qualifications and employment of nursing staff members.

_____

_____

_____ 9. Establishes and maintains an effective patient classification system.

_____

_____

_____ 10. Develops a system for evaluation of work performance and evaluates the performance of management personnel accordingly; sees that this system is maintained and that workers are evaluated in a fair and objective manner.

_____

_____

_____ 11. Plans ways to promote the growth and development of personnel through inservice programs, workshops, seminars, and other continuing education opportunities.

_____

_____

_____ 12. Assists in establishing and maintaining a safety, fire, and disaster program in cooperation with administration and safety committee and assures proper handling and emergency care of patients, personnel, and visitors involved in accidents.

_____

_____

_____ 13. Outlines and interprets to personnel Nursing Service's role in disaster planning.

_____

_____

_____ 14. Serves on committees including but not limited to: Department Head Meetings, Medical Staff Committee (serves as formal liaison with the Medical Staff), Hospital Quality Assurance Committee, Infection Control, Safety, Pharmacy and Therapeutics, Medical Records, Institutional Planning Meetings, Nursing Education Committee, Nursing Quality Assurance, Nursing Policy and Procedure Committee, and Library Committee; attends hospital board meetings to represent Nursing Service; attends nursing staff meetings and inservice education meetings.

_____

_____

_____ 15. Plans ways to improve leadership skills and to anticipate and minimize problems, and ways to identify these problems and to plan their resolution.

_____

_____

III. *Implementation:*

_____ 1. Directs the formulation and implementation of policies, procedures, and standards of practice.

_____

_____

_____ 2. Conducts monthly management meetings.

_____

_____

_____ 3. Meets regularly with the Administrator to discuss objectives, staffing needs, budget, hospital policies, and management problems.

_____

_____

_____ 4. Maintains compliance with nursing care standards, hospital policies and procedures, and regulatory agency requirements.

_____

_____

_____ 5. Interprets nursing to hospital administration, medical staff, and related public.

_____

_____

_____ 6. Interprets policies, procedures, objectives, standards, philosophy, and other matters to personnel.

_____

_____

_____ 7. Interviews applicants for nursing positions, approves applicants for hiring, and terminates employment of personnel when necessary.

_____

_____

_____ 8. Implements activities necessary to meet nursing objectives, as well as self-objectives.

_____

_____

_____ 9. Promotes harmonious relationships and favorable attitudes among the health care team.

_____

_____

_____ 10. Serves as consultant and role model for nursing personnel.

_____

_____

_____ 11. Initiates planned change and evaluates outcome to ensure that care is safe, efficient, and therapeutic.

_____

_____

_____ 12. In collaboration with Inservice Director, orients, instructs, and trains new personnel in nursing functions, policies, and procedures.

_____

_____

_____ 13. Assists and supports Inservice Director in conducting regular inservice meetings and in providing continuing education for personnel.

_____

_____

_____ 14. Ensures that regular staff meetings are held for all levels of personnel.

_____

_____

_____ 15. Establishes a system of record keeping and keeps personnel records current.

_____

_____

_____ 16. Maintains direct patient contact and involvement in patient care.

_____

_____

_____ 17. Investigates problems, irregularities, and policy violations and takes corrective action and follow-up when necessary.

_____

_____

_____ 18. Serves as consultant on hospital admitting and discharge procedures and other matters that affect patient care (or nursing service).

_____

_____

_____ 19. Prepares and submits budget information to administration.

_____

_____

_____ 20. Ensures that management personnel: provide unit orientation, education, and meetings on a regular basis; evaluate personnel; assess supply and equipment needs and maintain adequate stock of supplies.

_____

_____

_____ 21. Assists management personnel: in developing patient care plans and supervising other personnel in this area; in providing for psychosocial and spiritual needs of the patients; in helping unit personnel to maintain good mental, physical, and psychological health; in solving grievances and problems.

_____

_____

_____ 22. Assists management personnel in developing objectives, planned change, policy and procedure development, and in monitoring of standards of nursing care.

_____

_____

_____ 23. Keeps informed and up-to-date in all aspects of nursing care and management through literature, workshops, seminars, courses, and conferences with other nursing directors.

_____

_____

_____ 24. Maintains adequate reference library available to nursing personnel.

_____

_____

_____ 25. Maintains contact and communication with Administrator, department heads, and medical staff concerning all areas of direct and indirect patient care and hospital matters.

_____

_____

—————— 26. Conforms to hospital dress code.

———

———

—————— 27. Is rarely sick or absent from work due to health.

———

———

IV. *Evaluation:*

—————— 1. Evaluates and submits a report monthly concerning the functioning and progress of Nursing Service. Submits evaluation of achievement of goals and objectives, accomplishments, problems, and unusual happenings to the Administrator.

———

———

—————— 2. Evaluates and analyzes incident reports and takes the appropriate follow-up action.

———

———

—————— 3. Continually evaluates the care delivered by regular review of management reports, direct observation and patient rounds, results for quality assurance studies, review of charts and care plans, results of monitory standards, patient questionnaires, and by other sources. Ensures continual corrective and follow-up action where deficient.

———

———

—————— 4. Evaluates and revises goals and objectives as well as self-objectives.

———

———

—————— 5. Evaluates the performance of supervisors and head nurses according to their job descriptions.

———

———

—————— 6. Evaluates patient classification and staffing on a regular basis and revises as necessary.

———

———

_____ 7. Evaluates and revises forms to be used in nursing department or that affect Nursing Service.

_____

_____

_____ 8. Evaluates facilities and equipment used in the department.

_____

_____

_____ 9. Oversees actions of Nursing Quality Assurance Committee and sees that all pertinent information is related to the hospital-wide Quality Assurance Program.

_____

_____

_____ 10. Evaluates and revises policies and procedures.

_____

_____

_____ 11. Evaluates the effectiveness of problem-solving techniques.

_____

_____

_____ 12. Evaluates personnel's performance during emergencies and hospital disasters.

_____

_____

_____ 13. Constantly evaluates attitudes, morale, and interpersonal relationships and promotes ways to improve in these areas.

_____

_____

_____ 14. Evaluates effectiveness of orientation and staff development programs.

_____

_____

_____ 15. Evaluates and ensures that nursing process is carried out in a continuous manner on all patients.

_____

_____

DIRECTOR OF NURSING SERVICE: SCORING PROCEDURE

Instructions: Total the number of each item and multiply times the appropriate number. Add these totals to make the score.

U _____ × 0 = _____

S _____ × 1 = _____

A _____ × 2 = _____

E _____ × 3 = _____   _____ Total Score

Compare total score to the following scale to determine rank:

U	S	A	E
0 to 55	56 to 98	99 to 148	149 to 186

Overall Performance Review Score _____.

ALL ITEMS IN THE FOLLOWING SECTION MUST BE COMPLETED:

A. Interviewer's comments on overall review _____

_____

_____

B. Additional suggestions for overall work improvement and goals for next evaluation _____

_____

_____

C. Self-objectives _____

_____

_____

_____

_____   _____
Date   Employee's signature

_____   _____
Date   Administrator

DIRECTOR OF INSERVICE EDUCATION: JOB DESCRIPTION

Position Requirements:	Graduate from an accredited school of nursing with current licensure as a registered nurse in the State of Alabama. Three years experience in various phases of clinical nursing practice and adult education. A Bachelor's Degree is preferred. Awareness of current concepts of health care and community resources.
Professional Requirements:	Pursues programs of continuing education consistent with requirements of the Alabama Nurses' Association. Participates in educational conferences and updates and maintains professional knowledge and skills related to the management of areas of responsibility.
Position Accountable to:	Director of Nursing.
Position Summary:	Under the general supervision of the Director of Nursing Service, the Inservice Education Director's primary function is to assess, plan, implement, and evaluate the educational programs for Nursing Service. To plan patient education programs and to provide and promote appropriate orientation programs for all new nursing service employees.

I. *Assessment*
  1. Assesses the educational and performance needs of employees in collaboration with the Director of Nursing, Supervisors, and other personnel.
  2. Participates with Director of Nursing in assessing data concerning the overall operation of Nursing Service activities and the quality of patient care.
  3. Participates with Infection Control Nurse in assessing infection control practices and need for improvement.
  4. Assesses and evaluates research findings for application into inservice and continuing education programs.
  5. Assesses, plans, implements, and evaluates patient education programs.

II. *Planning*
  1. Formulates inservice education objectives in accordance with the philosophy and objectives of Nursing Service.
  2. Establishes criteria for all inservice education programs, constructing the curriculum, course outlines, objectives, teaching methods, examinations, and evaluation tools for each program.

3. Plans and develops self-objectives.
4. Participates with Director of Nursing in planning problem-solving techniques and ways to make improvements in Nursing Service.
5. Plans, organizes, and utilizes the resources and facilities available to accomplish the objectives of the department.
6. Participates with the Director of Nursing in budget planning, which provides for necessary human and environmental resources to achieve inservice objectives.
7. Contributes to the development of philosophy, goals and objectives, policies and procedures, and job descriptions in the institution.

III. *Implementation*

1. Plans and implements an orientation program for all Nursing Service personnel and provides for individualized counseling and guidance for educational needs or deficits.
2. Supplements and integrates inservice education into everyday practice.
3. Utilizes theories of leadership and methods of instruction in such a manner as to encourage and foster participation, cooperation, and motivation to learn.
4. Utilizes educational opportunities outside the hospital in order to meet the identified learning needs of the employees.
5. Provides professional literature and current periodicals to hospital personnel in order to foster continuing updating of knowledge.
6. Serves as a resource person and consultant to any hospital employee in order to provide ongoing learning and self-improvement.
7. Participates and promotes membership, interest, and active involvement in the activities of the professional organizations, in health care and community services, and in supportive community endeavors.
8. Participates in all activities that further professional growth and development.
9. Prepares an annual report of the Inservice Education Department including evaluation, necessary revisions, and recommendations and rationale for future learning experiences.
10. Has thorough knowledge of hospital policies and objectives and the ability to interpret this knowledge to personnel, to patients and their families, and to the community.
11. Understands the legal, social, economic, and political forces that influence the health care delivery system; keeps abreast of new legislation and regulations that affect standards of nursing practice and patient care.
12. By example and teaching, instills in each employee an appreciation of individual contribution in delivering the optimum quality care in the institution.
13. Assists in the supervision of personnel to ensure continuity of achievement of educational and hospital goals and objectives.

14. Assists in ensuring Nursing Service compliance with Joint Commission Standards, as well as Nursing Service Standards of Practice.
15. Engages in clinical practice to maintain clinical skills and expertise.
16. Serves on committees as requested.
17. Serves as chairperson of the Nursing Education Committee.
18. Conforms to hospital dress code.
19. Is rarely sick or absent from work due to health.

IV. *Evaluation*

1. Evaluates educational experiences designed to meet the assessed needs of all personnel, in cooperation and consultation with the Director of Nursing and Supervisors.
2. Formulates and implements tools for evaluation and methods of follow-up study for the orientation, inservice education, and continuing education programs.
3. Develops, maintains, and reviews records and reports pertinent to the inservice education program in order to identify employee achievement and to provide data for evaluation.
4. Evaluates and submits monthly report concerning inservice education activities.
5. Evaluates and revises inservice as well as self-objectives.
6. Participates in evaluation and revision of forms used in nursing service.

DIRECTOR OF INSERVICE EDUCATION: PERFORMANCE EVALUATION

Name _____ Employment Date _____

Rating Period _____ To _____

Department _____ Job Title _____

Instructions: Using the following rating scale, indicate the quality of performance by placing the appropriate letter on the line to the left of the item.

U* – Unsatisfactory (does not meet job requirements)
S – Satisfactory (meets job requirements)
A – Above average (exceeds job requirements)
E* – Exceptional performance

I. *Assessment:*

_____ 1. Assesses the educational and performance needs of employees in collaboration with the Director of Nursing, supervisors, and other personnel.

_____

_____

_____ 2. Participates with Director of Nursing in assessing data concerning the overall operation of Nursing Service activities and the quality of patient care.

_____

_____

_____ 3. Participates with Infection Control Nurse in assessing infection control practices and need for improvement.

_____

_____

_____ 4. Assesses and evaluates research findings for application into inservice and continuing education programs.

_____

_____

*The evaluator is expected to comment on all items rated "U" or "E."

_____ 5. Assesses, plans, implements, and evaluates patient education programs.

_____

_____

II. *Planning:*

_____ 1. Formulates inservice education objectives in accordance with the philosophy and objectives of Nursing Service.

_____

_____

_____ 2. Establishes criteria for all inservice education programs, constructing the curriculum, course outlines, objectives, teaching methods, examinations, and evaluation tools for each program.

_____

_____

_____ 3. Plans and develops self-objectives.

_____

_____

_____ 4. Participates with Director of Nursing in planning problem-solving techniques and ways to make improvements in Nursing Service.

_____

_____

_____ 5. Plans, organizes, and utilizes the resources and facilities available to accomplish the objectives of the department.

_____

_____

_____ 6. Participates with the Director of Nursing in budget planning, which provides for necessary human and environmental resources to achieve inservice objectives.

_____

_____

_____ 7. Contributes to the development of philosophy, goals and objectives, policies and procedures, and job descriptions in the institution.

_____

_____

III. *Implementation:*

_____ 1. Plans and implements an orientation program for all Nursing Service personnel and provides for individualized counseling and guidance for educational needs or deficits.

_____

_____

_____ 2. Supplements and integrates inservice education into everyday practice.

_____

_____

_____ 3. Utilizes theories of leadership and methods of instruction in such a manner as to encourage and foster participation, cooperation, and motivation to learn.

_____

_____

_____ 4. Utilizes educational opportunities outside the hospital in order to meet the identified learning needs of the employees.

_____

_____

_____ 5. Provides professional literature and current periodicals to hospital personnel in order to foster continuing updating of knowledge.

_____

_____

_____ 6. Serves as a resource person and consultant to any hospital employee in order to provide ongoing learning and self-improvement.

_____

_____

_____ 7. Participates and promotes membership, interest, and active involvement in the activities of the professional organizations, in health care and community services and in supportive community endeavors.

_____

_____

_____ 8. Participates in all activities that further professional growth and development.

_____

_____

_____ 9. Prepares an annual report of the Inservice Education Department including evaluation, necessary revisions, and recommendations and rationale for future learning experiences.

_____

_____ 10. Has thorough knowledge of hospital policies and objectives and the ability to interpret this knowledge to personnel, patients and their families, and to the community.

_____

_____ 11. Understands the legal, social, economic, and political forces that influence the health care delivery system; keeps abreast of new legislation and regulations that affect standards of nursing practice and patient care.

_____

_____ 12. By example and teaching, instills in each employee an appreciation of individual contribution in delivering the optimum quality care in the institution.

_____

_____ 13. Assists in the supervision of personnel to ensure continuity of achievement of educational and hospital goals and objectives.

_____

_____ 14. Assists in ensuring Nursing Service compliance with Joint Commission Standards, as well as Nursing Service Standards of Practice.

_____

_____ 15. Engages in clinical practice to maintain clinical skills and expertise.

_____

_____ 16. Serves on committees as requested.

_____

_____ 17. Serves as chairperson of the Nursing Education Committee.

_____

_____ 18. Conforms to hospital dress code.

_____

_____

_____ 19. Is rarely sick or absent from work due to health.

_____

_____

IV. *Evaluation:*

_____ 1. Evaluates educational experiences designed to meet the assessed needs of all personnel in cooperation and consultation with the Director of Nursing and Supervisors.

_____

_____

_____ 2. Formulates and implements tools for evaluation and methods of follow-up study for the orientation, inservice education, and continuing education programs.

_____

_____

_____ 3. Develops, maintains, and reviews records and reports pertinent to the inservice education program in order to identify employee achievement and to provide data for evaluation.

_____

_____

_____ 4. Evaluates and submits monthly reports concerning inservice education activities.

_____

_____

_____ 5. Evaluates and revises inservice as well as self-objectives.

_____

_____

_____ 6. Participates in evlauation and revision of forms used in Nursing Service.

_____

_____

DIRECTOR OF INSERVICE EDUCATION:
SCORING PROCEDURE

Instructions: Total the number of each item and multiply times the appropriate number. Add these totals to make the score.

U _____ × 0 = _____

S _____ × 1 = _____

A _____ × 2 = _____

E _____ × 3 = _____   _____ Total Score

Compare total score to the following scale to determine rank:

U	S	A	E
0 to 32	33 to 58	59 to 88	89 to 111

Overall Performance Review Score _____.

ALL ITEMS IN THE FOLLOWING SECTION MUST BE COMPLETED:

A. Interviewer's comments on overall review _____

_____

_____

B. Additional suggestions for overall work improvement and goals for next evaluation _____

_____

_____

C. Self-objectives _____

_____

_____

_____

_____   _____
Date   Employee's signature

_____   _____
Date   Interviewer's signature

_____   _____
Date   Director of Nursing

INFECTION CONTROL NURSE: JOB DESCRIPTION

Position Requirements: Must be a graduate of accredited school of nursing with current licensure in the State of Alabama. Must be a Registered Nurse with 2 years clinical experience in a hospital setting and a working knowledge of the principles of epidemiology and infectious disease.

Position Accountable for: All behavior described in the position description.

Position Accountable to: Director of Nursing Service

Position Summary: Under direction of Infection Control Committee and supervision of Director of Nursing Service, is responsible for providing surveillance throughout the hospital in order to identify, investigate, and record data concerning nosocomial infections; and is directly responsible for initiating infection control measures as directed by the Infection Control Committee.

I. *Assessment*
1. Assesses the delivery of nursing care throughout the hospital and determines compliance with infection control policies and procedures.
2. Assesses culture reports weekly to determine:
   a.   infections present
   b.   nosocomial infections
   c.   infections community acquired
3. Assesses the employee health program on a regular basis and determines potential or evident infections.
4. Assesses patients' temperature charts to identify possible infections.
5. Assesses all patients with potential sources of contaminants (Observes IV sites, Foley catheters, suture lines, etc.).

II. *Planning*
1. Plans problem-solving techniques and activities to decrease nosocomial infections and to improve quality of patient care.
2. In collaboration with Director of Nursing and other supervisory personnel, plans ways to implement new infection policies and procedures.
3. Participates with Inservice Education Director in planning classes and ensures infection control principles are included.
4. Plans and develops self-objectives.

III. *Implementation*

1. Attends Infection Control Committee meetings and provides a bi-monthly summary including the following:
   a. Records and reports of the number and type of infections identified since previous meeting,
   b. List of patients isolated,
   c. Report of spot cultures taken,
   d. Report of any problems encountered, including all areas of surveillance,
   e. Suggestions submitted by members of the health care team for improving infection control.
2. Implements activities necessary to meeting self-objectives.
3. Maintains records of all infections including the location, isolation, and general treatment of infections and related problems.
4. Ensures that cultures of environmental objects are taken (walls, floors, ice machines, vents) as well as personnel when appropriate.
5. Reports all communicable or contagious diseases to the Public Health officials on a regular basis.
6. Participates and contributes to a Unified Quality Assurance Program.
7. Keeps Director of Nursing informed on all reportable situations.
8. Develops and maintains the Infection Control Manual for the hospital.
9. Maintains adequate and up-to-date department library and resources.
10. Promotes the achievement of nursing service objectives.
11. Promotes harmonious relations and favorable attitudes among the health care team.
12. Attends required inservice programs.
13. Maintains current knowledge concerning principles of epidemiology and infection control, through current literature, attendance of workshops and seminars, and membership in professional organization.
14. Maintains communication with all department heads and supervisors concerning Infection Control activities.
15. Conforms to hospital dress code.
16. Is rarely sick or absent from work due to health.

IV. *Evaluation*

1. Evaluates self-objectives, revises and formulates new objectives.
2. Evaluates infection control manual and revises as appropriate.
3. Evaluates nursing service policies and procedures and recommends addition of infection control principles as appropriate.
4. Evaluates effectiveness of problem-solving techniques and infection control activities implemented to decrease nosocomial infections.
5. Participates in evaluation of inservice education programs.
6. Evaluates isolation procedure and revises as appropriate.
7. Evaluates communication systems and techniques, concerning present or potential infections, between self and nursing units for effectiveness and corrects any breakdown found.

INFECTION CONTROL NURSE: PERFORMANCE EVALUATION

Name ———————————————— Employment Date ——————————

Rating Period ———————————— To ——————————————————

Department —————————————— Job Title ——————————————

Instructions: Using the following rating scale, indicate the quality of performance by placing the appropriate letter on the line to the left of the item.

U* – Unsatisfactory (does not meet job requirements)
S – Satisfactory (meets job requirements)
A – Above average (exceeds job requirements)
E* – Exceptional performance

I. *Assessment:*

———— 1. Assesses the delivery of nursing care throughout the hospital and determines compliance with infection control policies and procedures.

————————————————————————————

————————————————————————————

———— 2. Assesses culture reports weekly to determine:
   a. infections present
   b. nosocomial infections
   c. infections community acquired

————————————————————————————

————————————————————————————

———— 3. Assesses the employee health program on a regular basis and determines potential or evident infections.

————————————————————————————

————————————————————————————

———— 4. Assesses patient's temperature charts to identify possible infections.

————————————————————————————

————————————————————————————

————————————————

*The evaluator is expected to comment on all items rated "U" or "E."

_____ 5. Assesses all patients with potential sources of contaminants (observes IV sites, Foley catheters, suture lines, etc.).

_____

_____

II. *Planning:*

_____ 1. Plans problem-solving techniques and activities to decrease nosocomial infections and improve quality of patient care.

_____

_____

_____ 2. In collaboration with Director of Nursing and other supervisory personnel, plans ways to implement new infection policies and procedures.

_____

_____

_____ 3. Participates with Inservice Education Director in planning classes and ensures Infection Control principles are included.

_____

_____

_____ 4. Plans and develops self-objectives.

_____

_____

III. *Implementation:*

       1. Attends Infection Control Committee meetings and provides a bi-monthly summary, including the following

_____ a. Records and reports of the number and type of infections identified since previous meeting.

_____

_____

_____ b. List of patients isolated.

_____

_____

_____ c. Report of spot cultures taken.

_____

_____

_____ d. Report of any problems encountered, including all areas of surveillance.

_____

_____

_____ e. Suggestions submitted by members of the health care team for improving infection control.

_____

_____

_____ 2. Implements activities necessary to meeting self-objectives.

_____

_____

_____ 3. Maintains records of all infections, including the location, isolation, and general treatment of infections and related problems.

_____

_____

_____ 4. Ensures that cultures of any environmental objects are taken (walls, floors, ice machines, vents) as well as personnel when appropriate.

_____

_____

_____ 5. Reports all communicable or contagious diseases to the public health officials on a regular basis.

_____

_____

_____ 6. Participates and contributes to a Unified Quality Assurance Program.

_____

_____

_____ 7. Keeps Director of Nursing informed on all reportable situations.

_____

_____

_____ 8. Develops and maintains the Infection Control Manual for the hospital.

_____

_____

_____ 9. Maintains adequate and up-to-date department library and resources.

_____

_____

_____ 10. Promotes the achievement of Nursing Service objectives.

_____

_____

_____ 11. Promotes harmonious relations and favorable attitudes among the health care team.

_____

_____

_____ 12. Attends required inservice programs.

_____

_____

_____ 13. Maintains current knowledge concerning principles of epidemiology and infection control through current literature, attendance of workshops and seminars, and membership in professional organization.

_____

_____

_____ 14. Maintains communication with all department heads and supervisors concerning Infection Control activities.

_____

_____

_____ 15. Conforms to hospital dress code.

_____

_____

_____ 16. Is rarely sick or absent from work due to health.

_____

_____

IV. *Evaluation:*

_____ 1. Evaluates self-objectives, revises and formulates new objectives.

_____

_____

_____ 2. Evaluates Infection Control Manual and revises as appropriate.

_____

_____

_____ 3. Evaluates Nursing Service policies and procedures and recommends addition of infection control principles as appropriate.

_____

_____

_____ 4. Evaluates effectiveness of problem-solving techniques and infection control activities implemented to decrease nosocomial infections.

_____

_____

_____ 5. Participates in evaluation of inservice education programs.

_____

_____

_____ 6. Evaluates isolation procedure and revises as appropriate.

_____

_____

_____ 7. Evaluates communication systems and techniques, concerning present or potential infections, between self and nursing units for effectiveness and corrects any breakdown found.

_____

_____

INFECTION CONTROL NURSE: SCORING PROCEDURE

Instructions: Total the number of each item and multiply times the appropriate number. Add these totals to make the score.

U _____ × 0 = _____

S _____ × 1 = _____

A _____ × 2 = _____

E _____ × 3 = _____   _____ Total Score

Compare total score to the following scale to determine rank:

U	S	A	E
0 to 31	32 to 57	58 to 85	86 to 108

Overall Performance Review Score _____.

ALL ITEMS IN THE FOLLOWING SECTION MUST BE COMPLETED:

A. Interviewer's comments on overall review _____

_____

_____

B. Additional suggestions for overall work improvement and goals for next evaluation _____

_____

_____

C. Self-objectives _____

_____

_____

_____

_____ Date

Employee's signature _____

_____ Date

Interviewer's signature _____

_____ Date

Director of Nursing _____

CENTRAL SERVICE SUPERVISOR: JOB DESCRIPTION

Position Requirements:	Graduate from an accredited school of nursing with current licensure as a registered nurse in the State of Alabama. Three years recent clinical experience in surgery, recovery room, or central services, including at least 1 year supervisory experience.
Professional Requirements:	Pursues programs of continuing education consistent with requirements of the Alabama Nurses' Association. Participates in educational conferences and updates and maintains professional knowledge and skills related to the management of areas of responsibility.
Position Accountable to:	Director of Nursing
Position Accountable for:	All behavior described in the Central Service Supervisor position description.
Position Summary:	Performs the primary functions of a professional leader in assessing, planning, directing, and evaluating Central Service activities on a 24-hour basis. Is responsible for meeting the Joint Commission Standards of Patient Care as well as established Nursing Service's Standards of Nursing Care, for managing all assigned personnel, supplies, and equipment in the unit, and for promoting teamwork with physicians and personnel of other departments.

I. *Assessment*
   1. Assesses the number and level of personnel needed to provide services and adjusts staffing appropriately.
   2. Assesses all Central Service activities, identifies problems and any need for improvement.
   3. Works with Nursing Staff and Central Service staff in promoting improvements in departmental and staff interactions.
   4. Makes a weekly assessment of all CSR machines (K-pads, gomco, suction) to ensure safety, proper cleaning, and tagging.

II. *Planning*
   1. Serves on hospital committees, helps plan programs, and revises and develops policies and procedures for department.
   2. Plans and develops self-objectives.

    3. Plans ways to solve problems and to make improvements in Central Service activities.

III. *Implementation*

    1. Implements activities necessary to meeting self-objectives.

    2. Promotes the achievement of nursing service objectives.

    3. Directs and implements planned changes and activities to improve Central Service department in collaboration with the Director of Nursing.

    4. Holds self and staff accountable for the delivery of quality of Central Service duties.

    5. Acts rapidly and effectively, follows hospital policies and procedures, and utilizes principles of management in any emergency situation.

    6. Promotes harmonious and favorable attitudes among the health care team.

    7. Assists with orientation of new employees in Central Service.

    8. Is knowledgeable of location, care, and operation of all equipment pertaining to Central Service.

    9. Keeps the Director of Nursing Service informed on reportable situations.

   10. Attends required inservice education programs.

   11. Serves as consultant in technical and professional matters for personnel.

   12. Participates and contributes to a unified Quality Assurance Program.

   13. Participates in the provision of inservice education programs for Central Service.

   14. Ensures that infection control policies and procedures are implemented properly.

   15. Ensures that all personnel are familiar with Central Service policies and procedures.

   16. Conforms to hospital dress code.

   17. Is rarely sick or absent from work due to health.

IV. *Evaluation*

    1. Continually evaluates Central Service activities by reviewing records, reports, charts, interviewing, observing, participating in Quality Assurance activities, and by employing other means of evaluation.

    2. Evaluates policies and procedures and revises as necessary in collaboration with Director of Nursing.

    3. Evaluates self-objectives and determines need for revision and new objectives.

    4. Evaluates the effectiveness of problem-solving techniques and activities.

    5. Evaluates the performance of Central Service personnel.

    6. Evaluates emergencies and any hospital disaster and recommends revisions in policies and procedures and/or need for improvement in Central Supply employee performance.

7. Evaluates orientation policies and procedures and recommends revisions as necessary.
8. Evaluates inservice education programs.
9. Evaluates autoclaved supplies and ensures that the procedure is implemented properly.
10. Evaluates supply charge system:
    a. Ensures that charges are made daily and logged properly.
    b. Receives feedback from the Business Office concerning problems and revises system appropriately.

CENTRAL SERVICE SUPERVISOR: PERFORMANCE EVALUATION

Name _____ Employment Date _____

Rating Period _____ To _____

Department _____ Job Title _____

Instructions: Using the following rating scale, indicate the quality of performance by placing the appropriate letter on the line to the left of the item.

U* – Unsatisfactory (does not meet job requirements)
S – Satisfactory (meets job requirements)
A – Above average (exceeds job requirements)
E* – Exceptional performance

I. *Assessment:*

_____ 1. Assesses the number and level of personnel needed to provide services and adjusts staffing appropriately.

_____

_____

_____ 2. Assesses all Central Service activities, identifies problems and any need for improvement.

_____

_____

_____ 3. Works with Nursing staff and Central Service staff in promoting improvements in departmental and staff interactions.

_____

_____

_____ 4. Makes a weekly assessment of all CSR machines (K-pads, gomco, suction) to ensure safety, proper cleaning, and tagging.

_____

_____

II. *Planning:*

_____ 1. Serves on hospital committees, helps plan programs, and revises and develops policies and procedures for department.

_____

_____

*The evaluator is expected to comment on all items rated "U" or "E."

_____ 2. Plans and develops self-objectives.

    _____

    _____

_____ 3. Plans ways to solve problems and to make improvements in Central Service activities.

    _____

    _____

III. _Implementation:_

_____ 1. Implements activities necessary to meeting self-objectives.

    _____

    _____

_____ 2. Promotes the achievement of Nursing Service objectives.

    _____

    _____

_____ 3. Directs and implements planned changes and activities to improve Central Service Department in collaboration with the Director of Nursing.

    _____

    _____

_____ 4. Holds self and staff accountable for the delivery of quality Central Service duties.

    _____

    _____

_____ 5. Acts rapidly and effectively, follows hospital policies and procedures, and utilizes principles of management in any emergency situation.

    _____

    _____

_____ 6. Promotes harmonious and favorable attitudes among the health care team.

    _____

    _____

_____ 7. Assists with orientation of new employees in Central Service.

    _____

    _____

_____ 8. Is knowledgeable of location, care, and operation of all equipment pertaining to Central Service.

_____

_____

_____ 9. Keeps the Director of Nursing Service informed on reportable situations.

_____

_____

_____ 10. Attends required inservice education programs.

_____

_____

_____ 11. Serves as consultant in technical and professional matters for personnel.

_____

_____

_____ 12. Participates and contributes to a unified Quality Assurance Program.

_____

_____

_____ 13. Participates in the provision of inservice education programs for Central Service.

_____

_____

_____ 14. Ensures that infection control policies and procedure are implemented properly.

_____

_____

_____ 15. Ensures that all personnel are familiar with Central Service policies and procedures.

_____

_____

_____ 16. Conforms to hospital dress code.

_____

_____

———— 17. Is rarely sick or absent from work due to health.

IV. *Evaluation:*

———— 1. Continually evaluates Central Service activities by reviewing records, reports, and charts, by interviewing, observing, and participating in Quality Assurance activities, and by employing other means of evaluation.

———— 2. Evaluates policies and procedures and revises as necessary in collaboration with Director of Nursing.

———— 3. Evaluates self-objectives and determines need for revision and new objectives.

———— 4. Evaluates the effectiveness of problem-solving techniques and activites.

———— 5. Evaluates the performance of Central Service personnel.

———— 6. Evaluates emergencies and any hospital disaster and recommends revisions in policies and procedures and/or need for improvement in Central Supply employee performance.

———— 7. Evaluates orientation policies and procedures and recommends revisions as necessary.

_____ 8. Evaluates inservice education programs.

_____

_____

_____ 9. Evaluates autoclaved supplies and ensures that the procedure is implemented properly.

_____

_____

_____ 10. Evaluates supply charge system:
   a. ensures that charges are made daily and logged properly,
   b. receives feedback from the business office concerning problems and revises system appropriately.

_____

_____

CENTRAL SERVICE SUPERVISOR: SCORING PROCEDURE

Instructions: Total the number of each item and multiply times the appropriate number. Add these totals to make the score.

U _____ ×0=_____

S _____ ×1=_____

A _____ ×2=_____

E _____ ×3=_____   _____ Total Score

Compare total score to the following scale to determine rank:

U	S	A	E
0 to 30	31 to 53	54 to 81	82 to 102

Overall Performance Review Score _____.

ALL ITEMS IN THE FOLLOWING SECTION MUST BE COMPLETED:

A. Interviewer's comments on overall review _____
_____
_____

B. Additional suggestions for overall work improvement and goals for next evaluation _____
_____
_____

C. Self-objectives _____
_____
_____
_____

_____ Date

_____ Date

_____ Date

_____ Employee's signature

_____ Interviewer's signature

_____ Director of Nursing

13

Task-Oriented Job Descriptions and Performance Evaluations

MEDICAL-SURGICAL NURSING ASSISTANT AND ORDERLY (DAY AND EVENING SHIFTS): JOB DESCRIPTION

Position Requirements:	Good physical and mental health. Minimum of grammar school education, high school or equivalent desirable. Genuine interest in welfare of the ill. Willingness to work under close supervision. Ability to follow written or verbal instructions effectively.
Position Accountable for:	All nursing care behaviors described in the position description.
Position Accountable to:	Licensed Practical Nurse, Registered Nurse in charge of unit, Head Nurse, Supervisor, Director of Nursing, patient, and family.
Position Summary:	Performs the functions of a nursing assistant in carrying out all assignments given by the Registered Nurse or Licensed Practical Nurse in charge of the unit. Is accountable for all patient care he/she gives during a shift. Is responsible for adhering to all Standards of Nursing Care and for promoting teamwork among co-workers.

RESPONSIBILITIES AND DUTIES

The Nursing Assistant shall provide the following for patients assigned to him/her:

1. Oral hygiene
2. a. AM care (bath-tub, shower, bed, etc.)
   b. PM care (back rub, etc.)
3. Sitz bath—as ordered
4. Provide clean linen when appropriate:
   a. Make unoccupied bed,
   b. Make occupied bed,
   c. Make postanesthetic bed,
   d. Change and straighten linen to remove wrinkles.
5. Give and remove bedpan/urinal.
6. Assist patients to and from bathroom.

The word *Nursing Assistant* is used interchangeably with *Orderly* in this job description. Orderlies perform duties relating to male patients only. Orderlies assist with female patients when asked or as indicated.

7. Positioning patients:
   a. Position patients according to RN's instructions (fowler's, semifowler's, etc.),
   b. Changes patient's position appropriately and as frequently as instructed.

8. Dietary needs:
   a. Ensure patient receives prescribed diet,
   b. Places tray conveniently for patient (on overbed table with head of bed up),
   c. Assist or feed patient as needed,
   d. Encourage good food intake to promote healing,
   e. Provide all snacks at ordered time (especially for diabetic patients, etc.),
   f. Remove tray and inform RN/LPN of patient's appetite (good, fair, poor, or refused),
   g. Provide fluids as instructed.

9. Intake and output:
   a. Post I & O sheet in room and I & O sign on door,
   b. Document on I & O sheet all intake and output for the shift, including gomco, suction, hemovac, T-tubes and Foley outputs,
   c. Turns I & O sheet in to RN/LPN 30 minutes prior to end of shift.

10. Specimen collection: The Nursing Assistant will obtain specimens according to the RN/LPN's instructions:
    a. Urine
    b. Sputum
    c. Stool
    d. 24-hour urine
    e. Clean catch urine
    f. Label all specimens with full name and time collected
    g. Take specimens to lab and clock in the time on lab slip.

11. Vital signs: The Nursing Assistant will take vital signs as instructed by RN or LPN. Included are:
    a. Temperature as ordered (orally, rectally, or axillary),
    b. Heart rate (pulse),
    c. Respiration Rate—Including description (rapid, shallow, deep, regular, or moist, etc.),
    d. Blood pressure,
    e. The Nursing Assistant will notify RN or LPN of any change or abnormal finding.

12. Treatments: The Nursing Assistant will be responsible for the following for patients assigned to him/her, as instructed by RN or LPN:
    a. Weigh patient
    b. Give enema
    c. Insert rectal tube
    d. Give perineal care
    e. Apply vaginal pads
    f. Test urine for sugar and acetone and notify RN of results immediately
    g. Apply hot or cold compresses
    h. Apply ice cap
    i. Apply ace bandages

    j. Give douche

    k. Care of body past death

13. The Nursing Assistant will assist RN or LPN with the following:

    a. Use of traction

    b. Use of restraints

    c. Observe IV

    d. Draping, examination, and treatment of patients

    e. Observe patients receiving blood for signs and symptoms of reaction

    f. Care of patient with:

        (1) Oxygen mask or cannula

        (2) Chest tubes

        (3) Foley catheter (urine meter, obtaining specimen, catheter care, and securing catheter bag to bed)

        (4) Colostomy

        (5) Hemovac drain

        (6) N.G. tube

        (7) Cast

        (8) Other duties as requested

14. Preoperative care:

    a. Ensure that side rails remain in up position and patient remains in bed past preoperative medication,

    b. Apply antiembolitic hose,

    c. Assist with moving patient from bed to stretcher.

15. Postoperatively assist RN or LPN as instructed: (i.e., turning, coughing, and deep breathing).

16. Admissions: The Nursing Assistant will be responsible for the following:

    a. Bringing patient to room from Admitting or Emergency Room,

    b. Assisting patient to bed and applying patient armband and name plate on door,

    c. Obtaining vital signs, height and weight, noting allergies, and reporting to RN or LPN,

    d. Assuring patient is comfortable and oriented to surroundings,

    e. Assisting RN or LPN with initial patient interview,

    f. Obtaining and explaining comfort kit.

17. Patient/family orientation—instruct/explain the following:

    a. Call signal

    b. Bed controls

    c. Thermostat

    d. Telephone

    e. T.V.

    f. Library

    g. Visitor policy

    h. Mealtimes

    i. Bathroom, showers, or bath

    j. Introduce room mate

    k. Smoking policy

    l. Side-rail policy

    m. Give information booklet

18. Discharge: The Nursing Assistant will be responsible for the following:
    a. Helping the patient collect personal belongings,
    b. Taking patient per wheelchair to car or lobby.

19. Transfers: The Nursing Assistant will:
    a. Collect patient's personal belongings,
    b. Assist patient to wheelchair or stretcher,
    c. Accompany patient to new room,
    d. Provide with call light and orient to new surroundings.

20. Comfort of patient: The Nursing Assistant is responsible for providing the following:
    a. patient privacy,
    b. skin care—keeps skin dry and clean, reports any noted reddened areas,
    c. straightening of patient's room,
    d. answering call lights promptly,
    e. additional comfort measures.

21. Equipment: The Nursing Assistant should be familiar with the following:
    a. care of orthopedic equipment,
    b. care of CSR equipment (suction, gomco, K-pads, etc),
    c. addressograph,
    d. any equipment necessary in performing his/her duties.

22. Safety:
    a. Ensures beds are in low position and locked at all times,
    b. Ensures that patients are secured appropriately when transporting by wheelchair or stretcher,
    c. Assists patients in moving, sitting, or ambulating as necessary,
    d. Ensures that needed articles are within patients' reach (water, tissues, bedpan, etc),
    e. Ensures that side rails remain in up position as indicated,
    f. Ensures that patient smoking policy is enforced,
    g. Ensures that patients remain restrained when necessary,
    h. Helps to ensure that the patient rooms remain free of clutter and pathway to bathroom is clear.

23. Is familiar with the operation and care of the following:
    a. CSR equipment (suction machines, K-pads, etc.)
    b. Orthopedic equipment

24. Infection control:
    a. Uses good handwashing and aseptic technique,
    b. Adheres to Isolation procedure,
    c. Helps to keep the unit clean,
    d. Gives Foley catheter care to patients daily.

25. Attends required inservice education programs, staff, and unit meetings.

26. Supports and adheres to Nursing Service and administrative policies and procedures.

27. Utilizes the aide check sheet as a means of reporting to RN or LPN.

28. Attends report and is prompt.

29. Cooperates and offers help to all personnel.

30. Answers all pages immediately.
31. Relates all patient questions/requests to nurse in charge.
32. Conforms to hospital dress code.
33. Is rarely sick or absent from work due to health.
34. Stays available and accessible at all times when on duty.

MEDICAL-SURGICAL NURSING ASSISTANT AND ORDERLY (DAY AND EVENING SHIFTS): PERFORMANCE EVALUATION

Name _____ Employment Date _____

Rating Period _____ To _____

Department _____ Job Title _____

Instructions: Using the following rating scale, indicate the quality of performance by placing the appropriate letter on the line to the left of the item.

U*– Unsatisfactory (does not meet job requirements)
S – Satisfactory (meets job requirements)
A – Above average (exceeds job requirements)
E* – Exceptional performance

RESPONSIBILITIES AND DUTIES

The Nursing Assistant shall provide the following for patients assigned to him/her:

_____ 1. Oral hygiene.

         _____

         _____

_____ 2. a. AM care (bath-tub, shower, bed, etc.)
            b. PM care (back rub, etc.)

         _____

         _____

_____ 3. Sitz bath—as ordered.

         _____

         _____

_____ 4. Provide clean linen when appropriate:
            a. Make unoccupied bed,
            b. Make occupied bed,
            c. Make postanesthetic bed,
            d. Change and straighten linen to remove wrinkles.

         _____

         _____

---

*The evaluator is expected to comment on all items rated "U" or "E."

_____ 5. Give and remove bedpan/urinal.

_____

_____

_____ 6. Assist patients to and from bathroom.

_____

_____

_____ 7. Positioning patients:
   a. Position patients according to RN's instructions (fowler's, semi-fowler's, etc.),
   b. Change patient's position appropriately and as frequently as instructed.

_____

_____

_____ 8. Dietary needs:
   a. Ensure patient receives prescribed diet,
   b. Place tray conveniently for patient (on overbed table with head of bed up),
   c. Assist or feed patient as needed,
   d. Encourage good food intake to promote healing,
   e. Provide all snacks at ordered time (especially for diabetic patients, etc.),
   f. Remove tray and inform RN/LPN of patient's appetite (good, fair, poor, or refused),
   g. Provide fluids as instructed.

_____

_____

_____ 9. Intake and Output:
   a. Post I & O sheet in room and I & O sign on door,
   b. Document on I & O sheet all intake and output for the shift, including gomco, suction, hemovac, T-tubes, and Foley outputs,
   c. Turn I & O sheet in to RN/LPN 60 minutes prior to end of shift.

_____

_____

_____ 10. Specimen collection: The Nursing Assistant will obtain specimens according to the RN/LPN's instructions:
   a. Urine
   b. Sputum
   c. Stool
   d. 24-hour urine
   e. Clean catch urine

     f. Label all specimens with full name and time collected,

     g. Take specimens to lab and clock in the time on lab slip.

_____ 11. Vital signs: The Nursing Assistant will take vital signs as instructed by the RN or LPN. Included are:

     a. Temperature as ordered (orally, rectally, or axillary),

     b. Heart rate (pulse),

     c. Respiration rate—including description (rapid, shallow, deep, regular, or moist, etc.),

     d. Blood pressure,

     e. The Nursing Assistant will notify RN or LPN of any change or abnormal finding.

_____ 12. Treatments: The Nursing Assistant will be responsible for the following for patients assigned to him/her, as instructed by RN or LPN:

     a. Weigh patient

     b. Give enema

     c. Insert rectal tube

     d. Give perineal care

     e. Apply vaginal pads

     f. Test urine for sugar and acetone and notify RN of results immediately

     g. Apply hot or cold compresses

     h. Apply ice cap

     i. Apply ace bandages

     j. Give douche

     k. Care of body past death

_____ 13. The Nursing Assistant will assist RN or LPN with the following:

     a. Use of traction,

     b. Use of restraints

     c. Observe IV

     d. Draping, examination, and treatment of patients

     e. Observe patients receiving blood for signs and symptoms of reaction

     f. Care of patient with:

        (1) Oxygen mask or cannula

        (2) Chest tubes

         (3) Foley catheter (urine meter, obtaining specimen, catheter care, and securing catheter bag to bed)
         (4) Colostomy
         (5) Hemovac drain
         (6) N. G. tube
         (7) Cast
         (8) Other duties as requested

_____

_____ 14. Preoperative care:
    a. Ensure that side rails remain in up position and patient remains in bed past preoperative medication,
    b. Apply antiembolitic hose,
    c. Assist with moving patient from bed to stretcher.

_____

_____ 15. Postoperatively assist RN or LPN as instructed (i.e., turning, coughing, and deep breathing).

_____

_____ 16. Admissions: The Nursing Assistant will be responsible for the following:
    a. Bringing patient to room from Admitting or Emergency Room,
    b. Assisting patient to bed and applying patient armband and name plate on door,
    c. Obtaining vital signs, height and weight, noting allergies, and reporting to RN or LPN,
    d. Assuring patient is comfortable and oriented to surroundings,
    e. Assisting RN or LPN with initial patient interview,
    f. Obtaining and explaining comfort kit.

_____

_____ 17. Patient/family orientation—instruct/explain the following:
    a. Call signal
    b. Bed controls
    c. Thermostat
    d. Telephone
    e. TV
    f. Library
    g. Visitor policy
    h. Mealtimes
    i. Bathroom, showers, or bath

    j. Introduce room mate

    k. Smoking policy

    l. Side rail policy

    m. Give information booklet

_____ 18. Discharge: The Nursing Assistant will be responsible for the following:

    a. Helping the patient collect personal belongings,

    b. Taking patient per wheelchair to car or lobby.

_____ 19. Transfers: The Nursing Assistant will:

    a. Collect patient's personal belongings,

    b. Assist patient to wheelchair or stretcher,

    c. Accompany patient to new room,

    d. Provide with call light and orient to new surroundings.

_____ 20. Comfort of patient: The Nursing Assistant is responsible for providing the following:

    a. Patient privacy,

    b. Skin care—keeps skin dry and clean, reports any noted reddened areas,

    c. Straightening of patient's room,

    d. Answering call lights promptly,

    e. Additional comfort measures.

_____ 21. Equipment: The Nursing Assistant should be familiar with the following:

    a. Care of orthopedic equipment,

    b. Care of CSR equipment (suction, gomco, K-pads, etc.),

    c. Addressograph,

    d. Any equipment necessary in performing his/her duties.

_____ 22. Safety:

    a. Ensures beds are in low position and locked at all times,

    b. Ensures that patients are secured appropriately when transporting by wheelchair or stretcher,

    c. Assists patients in moving, sitting, or ambulating as necessary,

    d. Ensures that needed articles are within patient's reach (water, tissues, bedpan, etc.),

    e. Ensures that side rails remain in up position as indicated,

    f. Ensures that patient smoking policy is enforced,

    g. Ensures that patients remain restrained when necessary,

    h. Helps to ensure that the patient rooms remain free of clutter and pathway to bathroom is clear.

_____ 23. Is familiar with the operation and care of the following:

    a. CSR equipment (suction machines, K-pads, etc.)

    b. Orthopedic equipment

_____ 24. Infection control:

    a. Uses good handwashing and aseptic technique,

    b. Adheres to isolation procedure,

    c. Helps to keep the unit clean,

    d. Gives Foley catheter care to patients daily.

_____ 25. Attends required inservice education programs, staff, and unit meetings.

_____ 26. Supports and adheres to Nursing Service and administrative policies and procedures.

_____ 27. Utilizes the aide check sheet as a means of reporting to RN or LPN.

_____ 28. Attends report and is prompt.

_____ 29. Cooperates and offers help to all personnel.

_____ 30. Answers all pages immediately.

_____

_____

_____ 31. Relates all patient questions/requests to nurse in charge.

_____

_____

_____ 32. Conforms to hospital dress code.

_____

_____

_____ 33. Is rarely sick or absent from work due to health.

_____

_____

_____ 34. Stays available and accessible at all times when on duty.

_____

_____

MEDICAL-SURGICAL NURSING ASSISTANT AND ORDERLY (DAY AND EVENING SHIFTS): SCORING PROCEDURE

Instructions: Total the number of each item and multiply times the appropriate number. Add these totals to make the score.

U _____ × 0 = _____

S _____ × 1 = _____

A _____ × 2 = _____

E _____ × 3 = _____   _____ Total Score

Compare total score to the following scale to determine rank:

U	S	A	E
0 to 30	31 to 53	54 to 81	82 to 102

Overall Performance Review Score _____.

ALL ITEMS IN THE FOLLOWING SECTION MUST BE COMPLETED:

A. Interviewer's comments on overall review _____
_____
_____

B. Additional suggestions for overall work improvement and goals for next evaluation _____
_____
_____

C. Self-objectives _____
_____
_____
_____

_____   _____
Date   Employee's signature

_____   _____
Date   Interviewer's signature

_____   _____
Date   Director of Nursing

MEDICAL-SURGICAL NURSING ASSISTANT AND ORDERLY (11 TO 7 SHIFT): JOB DESCRIPTION

Position Requirements: Good physical and mental health. Minimum of grammar school education, high school or equivalent desirable. Genuine interest in welfare of the ill. Willingness to work under close supervision. Ability to follow written or verbal instructions effectively.

Position Accountable for: All nursing care behaviors described in the position description.

Position Accountable to: Licensed Practical Nurse, Registered Nurse in charge of unit, Head Nurse, Supervisor, Director of Nursing, patient, and family.

Position Summary: Performs the functions of a nursing assistant in carrying out all assignments given by the Registered Nurse or Licensed Practical Nurse in charge of the unit. Is accountable for all patient care he/she gives during a shift. Is responsible for adhering to all Standards of Nursing Care and for promoting teamwork among co-workers.

RESPONSIBILITIES AND DUTIES

The Nursing Assistant shall provide the following for patients assigned to him/her:

1. Oral hygiene.
2. Provide clean linen when appropriate:
   a. making unoccupied bed,
   b. making occupied bed,
   c. making postanesthetic bed,
   d. change and straighten linen to remove wrinkles.
3. Give and remove bedpan/urinal.
4. Assist patients to and from bathroom.
5. Positioning patients:
   a. Position patient according to RN's instructions (fowler's, semifowler's, etc.),
   b. Change patients' position appropriately and as frequently as instructed.

The term *Nursing Assistant* is used interchangeably with *Orderly* in this job description. Orderlies perform duties relating to male patients only. Orderlies assist with female patients when asked or as indicated.

6. Dietary needs:
   a. Ensure patients are NPO as ordered,
   b. Ensure patients receive prescribed diet,
   c. Assist patient with food and fluids as needed,
   d. Provide fluids as instructed.

7. Intake and Output:
   a. Post I & O sheet in room and I & O sign on door,
   b. Document on I & O sheet all intake and output for the shift including gomco, suction, hemovac, T-tubes, and Foley outputs.

8. Specimen collection: The Nursing Assistant will obtain specimens according to the RN or LPN's instructions:
   a. Urine
   b. Sputum
   c. Stool
   d. 24-hour urine
   e. Clean catch urine
   f. Label all specimens with full name and time collected,
   g. Take specimens to lab and clock in the time on lab slip.

9. Vital signs: The Nursing Assistant will take vital signs as instructed by RN or LPN. Included are:
   a. Temperature as ordered (orally, rectally, or axillary),
   b. Heart rate (pulse),
   c. Respiration Rate—including description (rapid, shallow, deep, regular, or moist, etc.),
   d. Blood pressure,
   e. The Nursing Assistant will notify RN or LPN of any change or abnormal finding.

10. Treatments: The Nursing Assistant will be responsible for the following for patients assigned to him/her, as instructed by RN or LPN:
    a. Weigh patient
    b. Give enema
    c. Insert rectal tube
    d. Give perineal care
    e. Apply vaginal pads
    f. Test urine for sugar and acetone and notify RN of results immediately
    g. Apply hot or cold compresses
    h. Apply ice cap
    i. Apply ace bandages
    j. Give douche
    k. Care of body past death

11. The Nursing Assistant will assist RN or LPN with the following:
    a. Use of traction
    b. Use of restraints
    c. Observe IV
    d. Observe patients receiving blood for signs and symptoms of reaction
    e. Draping, examination, and treatment of patients
    f. Care of patient with:
       (1) Oxygen mask or cannula
       (2) Chest tubes

   (3) Foley catheter (urine meter, obtaining specimen, catheter care, and securing catheter bag to bed)
   (4) Colostomy
   (5) Hemovac drain
   (6) N.G. tube
   (7) Cast
   (8) Other duties as requested
12. Preoperative care:
    a. Ensure side rails remain in up position and patient remains in bed past preoperative medication,
    b. Apply antiembolitic hose,
    c. Assist with moving patient from bed to stretcher.
13. Postoperatively assists RN or LPN as instructed: (i.e., turning, coughing, and deep breathing).
14. Admissions: The Nursing Assistant will be responsible for the following:
    a. Bringing patient to room from Admitting or Emergency Room,
    b. Assisting patient to bed and applying patient armband and name plate on door,
    c. Obtaining vital signs, height and weight, noting allergies, and reporting to RN or LPN,
    d. Assuring patient is comfortable and oriented to surroundings,
    e. Assisting RN or LPN with initial patient interview,
    f. Obtaining and explaining comfort kit.
15. Patient/family orientation—instruct/explain the following:
    a. Call signal
    b. Bed controls
    c. Thermostat
    d. Telephone
    e. T.V.
    f. Library
    g. Visitor policy
    h. Mealtimes
    i. Bathroom, showers, bath
    j. Introduce to room mate
    k. Smoking policy
    l. Siderail policy
    m. Give information booklet
16. Transfers: The Nursing Assistant will:
    a. Collect patient's personal belongings,
    b. Assist patient to wheelchair or stretcher,
    c. Accompany patient to new room,
    d. Provide with call light and orient to new surroundings.
17. Comfort of patient: The Nursing Assistant is responsible for providing the following:
    a. Patient privacy,
    b. Skin care,
    c. Straightening of patient's room,
    d. Answering call lights promptly,
    e. Additional comfort measures.

18. Equipment: The Nursing Assistant should be familiar with the following:
    a. Care of orthopedic equipment,
    b. Care of CSR equipment,
    c. Addressograph,
    d. Any equipment necessary in performing his/her duties.

19. Safety:
    a. Ensures that beds are in low position and locked at all times,
    b. Ensures that patients are secured appropriately when transporting by wheelchair or stretcher,
    c. Assists patients in moving, sitting, or ambulating as necessary,
    d. Ensures that needed articles are within patient's reach (water, tissues, bedpan, etc.),
    e. Ensures that side rails remain in up position as indicated,
    f. Ensures that patient smoking policy is enforced,
    g. Ensures that patients remain restrained when necessary,
    h. Helps to ensure that patient's room remains free of clutter and pathway to bathroom is clear.

20. Is familiar with the operation and care of the following:
    a. CSR equipment (suction machines, K-pads, etc.)
    b. Orthopedic equipment

21. Infection control:
    a. Uses good handwashing and aseptic technique,
    b. Adheres to Isolation procedure and policies,
    c. Gives Foley catheter care to patients daily,
    d. Helps to keep the unit clean.

22. Attends inservice education programs, staff, and unit meetings.

23. Supports and adheres to Nursing Service and administrative policies and procedures.

24. Utilizes the aide check sheet as a means of reporting to RN or LPN.

25. Attends report and is prompt.

26. Cooperates and offers help to all personnel.

27. Answers all pages immediately.

28. Relates all patient questions/requests to nurse in charge.

29. Conforms to hospital dress code.

30. Is rarely sick or absent from work due to health.

31. Stays available and accessible at all times when on duty.

MEDICAL-SURGICAL NURSING ASSISTANT AND ORDERLY (11 TO 7 SHIFT): PERFORMANCE EVALUATION

Name _____ Employment Date _____

Rating Period _____ To _____

Department _____ Job Title _____

Instructions: Using the following rating scale, indicate the quality of performance by placing the appropriate letter on the line to the left of the item.

U*– Unsatisfactory (does not meet job requirements)
S – Satisfactory (meets job requirements)
A – Above average (exceeds job requirements)
E* – Exceptional performance

RESPONSIBILITIES AND DUTIES

The Nursing Assistant shall provide the following for patients assigned to him/her:

_____ 1. Oral hygiene.

          _____

          _____

_____ 2. Provides clean linen when appropriate:
        a. Makes unoccupied bed,
        b. Makes occupied bed,
        c. Makes postanesthetic bed,
        d. Changes and straightens linen to remove wrinkles.

          _____

          _____

_____ 3. Give and remove bedpan/urinal.

          _____

          _____

_____ 4. Assist patients to and from bathroom.

          _____

          _____

*The evaluator is expected to comment on all items rated "U" or "E."

_____ 5. Positioning patients:
   a. Position patient according to RN's instructions (fowler's, semi-fowler's, etc.),
   b. Change patient's position appropriately and as frequently as instructed.

_____

_____

_____ 6. Dietary needs:
   a. Ensure patients are NPO as ordered,
   b. Ensure patients receive prescribed diet,
   c. Assist patient with food and fluids as needed,
   d. Provide fluids as instructed.

_____

_____

_____ 7. Intake and Output:
   a. Post I & O sheet in room and I & O sign on door,
   b. Document on I & O sheet all intake and output for the shift, including gomco, suction, hemovac, T-tubes, and Foley outputs.

_____

_____

_____ 8. Specimen collection: The Nursing Assistant will obtain specimens according to the RN or LPN's instructions:
   a. Urine
   b. Sputum
   c. Stool
   d. 24-hour urine
   e. Clean catch urine
   f. Label all specimens with full name and time collected,
   g. Take specimens to lab and clock in the time on lab slip.

_____

_____

_____ 9. Vital signs: The Nursing Assistant will take vital signs as instructed by RN or LPN. Included are:
   a. Temperature as ordered (orally, rectally, or axillary),
   b. Heart rate (pulse),
   c. Respiration rate—including description (rapid, shallow, deep, regular, or moist, etc.),
   d. Blood pressure,
   e. The Nursing Assistant will notify RN or LPN of any change or abnormal finding.

_____

_____

_____ 10. Treatments: The Nursing Assistant will be responsible for the following for patients assigned to him/her, as instructed by RN or LPN:
   a. Weigh patient
   b. Give enema
   c. Insert rectal tube
   d. Give perineal care
   e. Apply vaginal pads
   f. Test urine for sugar and acetone and notify RN of results immediately
   g. Apply hot or cold compresses
   h. Apply ice cap
   i. Apply ace bandages
   j. Give douche
   k. Care of body past death

_____

_____

_____ 11. The Nursing Assistant will assist RN or LPN with the following:
   a. Use of traction
   b. Use of restraints
   c. Observe IV
   d. Observe patients receiving blood for signs and symptoms of reaction
   e. Draping, examination, and treatment of patients
   f. Care of patient with:
      (1) Oxygen mask or cannula
      (2) Chest tubes
      (3) Foley catheter (urine meter, obtaining specimen, catheter care, and securing catheter bag to bed)
      (4) Colostomy
      (5) Hemovac drain
      (6) N.G. tube
      (7) Cast
      (8) Other duties as requested

_____

_____

_____ 12. Preoperative care:
   a. Ensure side rails remain in up position and patient remains in bed past preoperative medication,
   b. Apply antiembolitic hose,
   c. Assist with moving patient from bed to stretcher.

_____

_____

_____ 13. Postoperatively assists RN or LPN as instructed (i.e., turning, coughing, and deep breathing).

_____

_____

_____ 14. Admissions: The Nursing Assistant will be responsible for the following:
   a. Bringing patient to room from Admitting or Emergency Room,
   b. Assisting patient to bed and applying patient armband and name plate on door,
   c. Obtaining vital signs, height and weight, noting allergies, and reporting to RN or LPN,
   d. Assuring patient is comfortable and oriented to surroundings,
   e. Assisting RN or LPN with initial patient interview,
   f. Obtaining and explaining comfort kit.

_____

_____

_____ 15. Patient/family orientation—instruct/explain the following:
   a. Call signal
   b. Bed controls
   c. Thermostat
   d. Telephone
   e. TV
   f. Library
   g. Visitor policy
   h. Mealtimes
   i. Bathroom, showers, bath
   j. Introduce to room mate
   k. Smoking policy
   l. Side rail policy
   m. Give information booklet

_____

_____

_____ 16. Transfers: The Nursing Assistant will:
   a. Collect patient's personal belongings,
   b. Assist patient to wheelchair or stretcher,
   c. Accompany patient to new room,
   d. Provide with call light and orient to new surroundings.

_____

_____

_____ 17. Comfort of patient: The Nursing Assistant is reponsible for providing the following:
   a. Patient privacy

    b. Skin care

    c. Straightening of patient's room

    e. Answering call lights promptly

    f. Additional comfort measures

_____ 18. Equipment: The Nursing Assistant should be familiar with the following:

    a. Care of orthopedic equipment

    b. Care of CSR equipment

    c. Addressograph

    d. Any equipment necessary in performing his/her duties

_____ 19. Safety:

    a. Ensures that beds are in low position and locked at all times,

    b. Ensures that patients are secured appropriately when transporting by wheelchair or stretcher,

    c. Assists patients in moving, sitting, or ambulating as necessary,

    d. Ensures that needed articles are within patient's reach (water, tissues, bedpan, etc.),

    e. Ensures that side rails remain in up position as indicated,

    f. Ensures that patient smoking policy is enforced,

    g. Ensures that patients remain restrained when necessary,

    h. Helps to ensure that patient's room remains free of clutter and pathway to bathroom is clear.

_____ 20. Is familiar with the operation and care of the following:

    a. CSR equipment (suction machines, K-pads, etc.)

    b. Orthopedic equipment

_____ 21. Infection control:

    a. Uses good handwashing and aseptic technique,

    b. Adheres to isolation procedure and policies,

    c. Gives Foley catheter care to patients daily,

    d. Helps to keep the unit clean.

_____ 22. Attends inservice education programs, staff, and unit meetings.

_____

_____

_____ 23. Supports and adheres to Nursing Service and administrative policies and procedures.

_____

_____

_____ 24. Utilizes the aide check sheet as a means of reporting to RN or LPN.

_____

_____

_____ 25. Attends report and is prompt.

_____

_____

_____ 26. Cooperates and offers help to all personnel.

_____

_____

_____ 27. Answers all pages immediately.

_____

_____

_____ 28. Relates all patient questions/requests to nurse in charge.

_____

_____

_____ 29. Conforms to hospital dress code.

_____

_____

_____ 30. Is rarely sick or absent from work due to health.

_____

_____

_____ 31. Stays available and accessible at all times when on duty.

_____

_____

MEDICAL-SURGICAL NURSING ASSISTANT AND ORDERLY (11 TO 7 SHIFT): SCORING PROCEDURE

Instructions: Total the number of each item and multiply times the appropriate number. Add these totals to make the score.

U _____ × 0 = _____

S _____ × 1 = _____

A _____ × 2 = _____

E _____ × 3 = _____   _____ Total Score

Compare total score to the following scale to determine rank:

U	S	A	E
0 to 27	28 to 49	50 to 73	74 to 93

Overall Performance Review Score _____.

ALL ITEMS IN THE FOLLOWING SECTION MUST BE COMPLETED:

A. Interviewer's comments on overall review _____
_____
_____

B. Additional suggestions for overall work improvement and goals for next evaluation _____
_____
_____

C. Self-objectives _____
_____
_____

_____   _____
Date   Employee's signature

_____   _____
Date   Interviewer's signature

_____   _____
Date   Director of Nursing

NURSING ASSISTANT—INTENSIVE AND CORONARY CARE UNIT: JOB DESCRIPTION

Position Requirements:	Good physical and mental health. Minimum of grammar school education, high school or equivalent desirable. Genuine interest in welfare of the ill. Willingness to work under close supervision. Ability to follow written or verbal instructions effectively. Specific Intensive and Coronary Care Unit orientation and training.
Position Accountable for:	All nursing care behaviors described in the position description.
Position Accountable to:	Registered Nurse in charge of unit, Head Nurse, Supervisor, Director of Nursing, patient, and family.
Position Summary:	Performs the functions of a nursing assistant in carrying out all assignments given by the Registered Nurse in charge of the unit. Is accountable for all patient care she gives during a shift. Is responsible for adhering to all Standards of Nursing Care and for promoting teamwork among co-workers.

RESPONSIBILITIES AND DUTIES

The Nursing Assistant shall provide the following for patients assigned to her:

1. Personal hygiene:
   a. oral hygiene
   b. AM care
   c. PM care (back rub, etc.)
   d. give and remove bedpan/urinal
2. Provides clean linen when appropriate:
   a. makes unoccupied bed
   b. makes occupied bed
   c. makes postanesthetic bed
   d. changes and straightens linen to remove wrinkles
3. Positioning patients:
   a. positions according to RN's instructions,
   b. Changes patient's position appropriately and as frequently as instructed.
4. Dietary needs:
   a. Ensures patients receive prescribed diets,
   b. Places tray conveniently for patient (on overbed table with head of bed up),

    c. Assists or feeds patients as needed,

    d. Encourages good food intake to promote healing,

    e. Provides all snacks at ordered time (especially for diabetic patients, etc.),

    f. Removes tray and informs RN of patient's appetite (good, fair, poor, or refused),

    g. Provides fluids as instructed.

5. Intake and Output:

    a. Posts I & O sheet and sign in room.

    b. Documents on I & O sheet all intake and output for the shift including gomco, suction, hemovac, T-tubes, and Foley outputs.

6. Specimen collection: Obtains specimens according to the RN's instructions:

    a. Urine

    b. Sputum

    c. Stool

    d. 24-hour urine

    e. Clean catch urine

    f. Labels all specimens with full name and time collected,

    g. Takes specimens to lab and clocks in the time on lab slip.

7. Vital signs: Takes vital signs as instructed by RN, including:

    a. Temperature as ordered (orally, rectally, or axillary),

    b. Heart rate (pulse),

    c. Respiration rate—including description (rapid, shallow, deep regular, or moist, etc.),

    d. Blood pressure,

    e. Notifies RN of any change or abnormal finding.

8. Treatments: Responsible for the following for patients assigned to her, as instructed by RN:

    a. Weigh patient

    b. Insert rectal tube

    c. Give enema

    d. Give perineal care

    e. Apply vaginal pads

    f. Test urine for sugar and acetone and notify RN of results immediately

    g. Apply hot or cold compresses

    h. Apply ice cap

    i. Apply ace bandages

    j. Give douche

    k. Care of body past death

9. Assists RN with the following:

    a. use of traction

    b. observe IV

    c. draping, examination, and treatment of patients

    d. observe patients receiving blood for signs and symptoms of reaction

    e. care of patient with:

        (1) Oxygen mask or cannula

        (2) Foley catheter (urine meter, obtaining specimen, catheter care, and securing catheter bag to bed)

        (3) Colostomy

        (4) Hemovac drain

(5) Cast

(6) Other duties as requested

10. Preoperative care:

a. Ensures side rails remain in up position and patient remains in bed past preoperative medication,

b. Applies antiembolitic hose,

c. Assists with moving patient from bed to stretcher.

11. Postoperatively assists RN as instructed (i.e., turning, coughing, and deep breathing).

12. Admissions: The Nursing Assistant will be responsible for the following:

a. Bringing patient to room from Admitting or Emergency Room,

b. Assisting patient to bed and applying patient armband,

c. Obtaining vital signs, height and weight, noting allergies, and reporting to RN,

d. Assuring patient is comfortable and oriented to surroundings,

e. Assisting RN with initial patient interview,

f. Obtaining and explaining comfort kit.

13. Patient/family orientation—instruct/explain the following:

a. Call signal

b. Library

c. Visitor policy

d. Mealtimes

e. Bath arrangements

f. Toilet arrangements

g. Side rail policy

14. Transfers: The Nursing Assistant will:

a. Collect patient's personal belongings,

b. Assist patient to wheelchair or stretcher,

c. Accompany patient to new room.

15. Comfort of patient: The Nursing Assistant is responsible for providing the following:

a. Patient privacy

b. Skin care (keeps patients clean and dry, reports any noted reddened areas)

c. Straightening of patient's room

d. Answering call lights promptly

e. Additional comfort measures

16. Safety:

a. Ensures beds are in low position and locked at all times,

b. Ensures that patients are secured appropriately when transported by wheelchair or stretcher,

c. Assists patients in moving, sitting, or ambulating as necessary,

d. Ensures that needed articles are within patients reach (water, tissues, bedpan, etc.),

e. Ensures that side rails remain in up position as indicated,

f. Ensures that patient smoking policy is enforced,

g. Ensures that patients remain restrained when necessary,

h. Helps to ensure that the unit remains clear of clutter and necessary supplies and equipment are accessible.
17. Is familiar with the operation and care of the following:
    a. CSR equipment (suction machines, K-pads, etc.)
    b. Orthopedic equipment
    c. Cardiac monitors
18. Infection control:
    a. Uses good handwashing and aseptic technique,
    b. Adheres to Isolation procedure,
    c. Helps to keep the unit clean,
    d. Gives Foley catheter care to patients daily.

Within the scope of the job description provides care for patients with the following:

    a. Central venous line
    b. Chest tube
    c. Pacemaker
    d. Rotating tourniquets
    e. N.G. tube
    f. Respirator
    g. Tracheostomy/endotracheal tube
19. Assists RN in caring for the dying patient.
20. Acts rapidly and calmly during emergencies and provides the necessary materials called for by the RN.
21. Stays available and accessible at all times when on duty.
22. Attends required inservice education programs, staff, and unit meetings.
23. Supports and adheres to Intensive and Coronary Care Unit and administrative policies and procedures.
24. Attends report and is prompt.
25. Relates all patient questions/requests to nurse in charge.
26. Conforms to hospital dress code.
27. Is rarely sick or absent from work due to health.

NURSING ASSISTANT—INTENSIVE AND CORONARY CARE UNIT: PERFORMANCE EVALUATION

Name _____ Employment date _____

Rating Period _____ To _____

Department _____ Job Title _____

Instructions: Using the following rating scale, indicate the quality of performance by placing the appropriate letter on the line to the left of the item.

U* – Unsatisfactory (does not meet job requirements)
S – Satisfactory (meets job requirements)
A – Above average (exceeds job requirements)
E* – Exceptional performance

RESPONSIBILITIES AND DUTIES

The Nursing Assistant shall provide the following for patients assigned to her:

_____ 1. Personal hygiene:
   a. Oral hygiene
   b. AM care
   c. PM care (back rub, etc.)
   d. Give and remove bedpan/urinal

   _____

   _____

_____ 2. Provides clean linen when appropriate:
   a. Makes unoccupied bed
   b. Makes occupied bed
   c. Makes postanesthetic bed
   d. Changes and straightens linen to remove wrinkles

   _____

   _____

_____

*The evaluator is expected to comment on all items rated "U" or "E."

350

_____ 3. Positioning patients:
   a. Positions according to RN's instructions,
   b. Changes patient's position appropriately and as frequently as instructed.

_____ 4. Dietary needs:
   a. Ensures patients receive prescribed diets,
   b. Places tray conveniently for patient (on overbed table with head of bed up),
   c. Assists or feeds patients as needed,
   d. Encourages good food intake to promote healing,
   e. Provides all snacks at ordered time (especially for diabetic patients, etc.),
   f. Removes tray and informs RN of patient's appetite (good, fair, poor, or refused),
   g. Provides fluids as instructed.

_____ 5. Intake and Output:
   a. Posts I & O sheet and signs in room,
   b. Documents on I & O sheet all intake and output for the shift, including gomco, suction, hemovac, T-tubes, and Foley outputs.

_____ 6. Specimen collection: Obtains specimens according to the RN's instructions:
   a. Urine
   b. Sputum
   c. Stool
   d. 24-hour urine
   e. Clean catch urine
   f. Label all specimens with full name and time collected
   g. Take specimens to lab and clock in the time on lab slip.

_____ 7. Vital signs: Takes vital signs as instructed by RN; included are:
   a. Temperature as ordered (orally, rectally, or axillary)
   b. Heart rate (pulse)

c. Respiration rate, including description (rapid, shallow, deep regular, or moist, etc.)
d. Blood pressure
e. Notifies RN of any change or abnormal finding.

_____

_____

_____ 8. Treatments: Responsible for the following for patients assigned to her, as instructed by RN:
   a. Weigh patient
   b. Insert rectal tube
   c. Give enema
   d. Give perineal care
   e. Apply vaginal pads
   f. Test urine for sugar and acetone and notify RN of results immediately
   g. Apply hot or cold compresses
   h. Apply ice cap
   i. Apply ace bandages
   j. Give douche
   k. Care of body past death

_____

_____

_____ 9. Assists RN with the following:
   a. Use of traction
   b. Observe IV
   c. Draping, examination, and treatment of patients
   d. Observe patients receiving blood for signs and symptoms of reaction
   e. Care of patients with:
      (1) Oxygen mask or cannula
      (2) Foley catheter (urine meter, obtaining specimen, catheter care, and securing catheter bag to bed)
      (3) Colostomy
      (4) Hemovac drain
      (5) Cast
      (6) Other duties as requested

_____

_____

_____ 10. Preoperative care:
   a. Ensures side rails remain in up position and patient remains in bed past preoperative medication,

    b. Applies antiembolitic hose,

    c. Assists with moving patient from bed to stretcher.

_____

_____

_____ 11. Postoperatively assists RN as instructed (i.e., turning, coughing, and deep breathing).

_____

_____

_____ 12. Admissions: The Nursing Assistant will be responsible for the following:

    a. Bringing patient to room from Admitting or Emergency Room,

    b. Assisting patient to bed and applying patient armband,

    c. Obtaining vital signs, height and weight, noting allergies, and reporting to RN,

    d. Assuring patient is comfortable and oriented to surroundings,

    e. Assisting RN with initial patient interview,

    f. Obtaining and explaining comfort kit.

_____

_____

_____ 13. Patient/family orientation—instruct/explain the following:

    a. Call signal

    b. Library

    c. Visitor policy

    d. Mealtimes

    e. Bath arrangements

    f. Toilet arrangements

    g. Side rail policy

_____

_____

_____ 14. Transfers: The Nursing Assistant will:

    a. Collect patient's personal belongings,

    b. Assist patient to wheelchair or stretcher,

    c. Accompany patient to new room.

_____

_____

_____ 15. Comfort of patient: The Nursing Assistant is responsible for providing the following:

    a. Patient privacy

    b. Skin care (keeps patients clean and dry, reports any noted reddened areas)

    c. Straightening of patient's room

    d. Answering call lights promptly

    e. Additional comfort measures

_____ 16. Safety:

    a. Ensures beds are in low position and locked at all times,

    b. Ensures that patients are secured appropriately when transported by wheelchair or stretcher,

    c. Assists patients in moving, sitting, or ambulating as necessary,

    d. Ensures that needed articles are within patient's reach (water, tissues, bedpan, etc.),

    e. Ensures that side rails remain in up position as indicated,

    f. Ensures that patient smoking policy is enforced,

    g. Ensures that patients remain restrained when necessary,

    h. Helps to ensure that the unit remains clear of clutter and necessary supplies and equipment are accessible.

_____ 17. Is familiar with the operation and care of the following:

    a. CSR equipment (suction machines, K-pads, etc.)

    b. Orthopedic equipment

    c. Cardiac monitors

_____ 18. Infection control:

    a. Uses good handwashing and aseptic technique,

    b. Adheres to isolation procedure,

    c. Helps to keep the unit clean,

    d. Gives Foley catheter care to patients daily.

Within the scope of the job description provides care for patients with the following:

_____ a. Central venous line

_____ b. Chest tube

_____ c. Pacemaker

_____

_____

_____ d. Rotating tourniquets

_____

_____

_____ e. N.G. tube

_____

_____

_____ f. Respirator

_____

_____

_____ g. Tracheostomy/endotracheal tube.

_____

_____

_____ 19. Assists RN in caring for the dying patient.

_____

_____

_____ 20. Acts rapidly and calmly during emergencies and provides the necessary materials called for by the RN.

_____

_____

_____ 21. Stays available and accessible at all times when on duty.

_____

_____

_____ 22. Attends required inservice education programs, staff, and unit meetings.

_____

_____

_____ 23. Supports and adheres to Intensive and Coronary Care Unit and administrative policies and procedures.

_____

_____

_____ 24. Attends report and is prompt.

_____

_____

_____ 25. Relates all patient questions/requests to nurse in charge.

_____

_____

_____ 26. Conforms to hospital dress code.

_____

_____

_____ 27. Is rarely sick or absent from work due to health.

_____

_____

NURSING ASSISTANT—INTENSIVE AND CORONARY CARE UNIT: SCORING PROCEDURE

Instructions: Total the number of each item and multiply times the appropriate number. Add these totals to make the score.

$$U \underline{\hspace{2cm}} \times 0 = \underline{\hspace{2cm}}$$
$$S \underline{\hspace{2cm}} \times 1 = \underline{\hspace{2cm}}$$
$$A \underline{\hspace{2cm}} \times 2 = \underline{\hspace{2cm}}$$
$$E \underline{\hspace{2cm}} \times 3 = \underline{\hspace{2cm}} \qquad \underline{\hspace{2cm}} \text{ Total Score}$$

Compare total score to the following scale to determine rank:

U	S	A	E
0 to 30	31 to 53	54 to 81	82 to 102

Overall Performance Review Score _____.

ALL ITEMS IN THE FOLLOWING SECTION MUST BE COMPLETED:

A. Interviewer's comments on overall review _____
_____
_____

B. Additional suggestions for overall work improvement and goals for next evaluation _____
_____
_____

C. Self-objectives _____
_____
_____
_____
_____

_____	_____
Date	Employee's signature
_____	_____
Date	Interviewer's signature
_____	_____
Date	Director of Nursing

EMERGENCY DEPARTMENT NURSING ASSISTANT AND ORDERLY: JOB DESCRIPTION

Position Requirements: Good physical and mental health. Minimum of grammar school education, high school or equivalent desirable. Genuine interest in welfare of ill. Willingness to work under close supervision. Ability to follow written or verbal instructions effectively. Specific orientation and training for Emergency Department.

Position Accountable for: All nursing care behaviors described in the position description.

Position Accountable to: RN in charge of Emergency Department, Director of Nursing, patient, and family.

Position Summary: Performs the functions of a nursing assistant in carrying out all assignments given by the RN in charge of Emergency Department. Is accountable for all patient care she/he gives in Emergency Department. Is responsible for adhering to all Standards of Nursing Care and for promoting teamwork among co-workers.

RESPONSIBILITIES AND DUTIES

Patient Admission to Emergency Department:

1. Assists patient from car with wheelchair or stretcher to Emergency Department, then to stretcher in examination room.
2. Assists with obtaining information from patient and/or family for Emergency Department records.
3. Obtains vital signs as directed by RN:
   a. Blood pressure
   b. Heart rate (pulse)
   c. Respiration rate (describe—rapid, shallow, regular, deep, etc.)
   d. Temperature (orally, axillary, or rectally)
4. Documents on designated portions of outpatient record.
5. Provides patient privacy.
6. Relates all patient/family questions to the RN.

Assists the RN as Instructed with:

7. Preparing patient for examination by physician
8. Cleaning patient in preparation for treatment
9. Draping and wrapping patient to maintain asepsis
10. Connecting patient to heart monitor

11. Safety of patient:
    a. Restrains as indicated,
    b. Ensure side rails are up when indicated,
    c. Assists patients in moving, sitting, and ambulating,
    d. Ensures patients are secured appropriately when transporting by wheel-chair or stretcher
12. Observing IV
13. Observing a patient receiving blood for signs and symptoms of reaction
14. Preop skin preparation
15. Application of casts by physician
16. Providing comfort measures
17. Intake and output
18. Oxygen therapy
19. Foley catheter (collecting specimens, securing bag, removing)

Assists RN in Caring for Patient with:
20. Central venous line
21. Chest tube
22. N.G. tube
23. Rotating tourniquets
24. Endotracheal tube/tracheostomy
25. Setting up sterile trays
26. Assists with specimen collection as requested:
    a. Urine—for U/A or clean catch
    b. Sputum
    c. Stool
    d. Other
    e. Label all specimens with patient's name, date, time, and source
    f. Take specimen to lab
27. Provides treatments as requested:
    a. Enema
    b. Insert Rectal tube
    c. Give perineal care
    d. Test urine for sugar and acetone
    e. Apply hot or cold compresses
    f. Apply ice cap
    g. Apply ace bandages
    h. Give bedpan/urinal
    i. Provide fluids as instructed
    j. Weighing patient
    k. Applying vaginal pads
28. Assists RN in completing Emergency Department charge tickets.
29. Requisitions lab and x-ray work.
30. Assists RN in running errands, making calls, xeroxing, etc.
31. Supports patient during:
    a. Electrocardiogram

    b. Lab and x-ray procedures

    c. Treatments

32. Assists with admission of patient from Emergency Department to room:

    a. Takes patient to room; directs family to admitting as requested,

    b. Assists patient from stretcher or wheelchair to bed,

    c. Assists patient in moving personal belongings to room,

    d. Orients patient to surroundings, assuring patient is comfortable,

    e. Provides call light, bedside needs, and explains how to call nurse,

    f. Gives nurses on floor any pertinent information concerning patient.

33. Is familiar with Emergency Department and administration policies and procedures.

34. Is familiar with contents of trays, packs, and the location of equipment and supplies.

35. Assists in patient discharge from Emergency Department:

    a. Assists patient with clothing and collecting personal belongings,

    b. Assists patient to car,

    c. Ensures that all forms and requisitions are completed before patient discharge,

    d. Cleans stretchers, and properly disposes of used supplies and equipment.

36. Is familiar with:

    a. All emergency equipment (Life Packs, MAST trousers, etc.),

    b. Care of orthopedic equipment,

    c. Care of CSR equipment and taking contaminated equipment back to CSR,

    d. Checks equipment for safety, proper operation, and tagging by maintenance.

37. Assists in maintaining ER supplies (Checks supplies and reorders as indicated).

38. Maintains confidentiality of patient information.

39. Demonstrates practice of infection control principles:

    a. handwashing

    b. aseptic technique

    c. sterile technique

    d. adheres to Isolation procedure

40. Acts rapidly and calmly during emergencies and provides necessary materials called for by the RN.

41. Cooperates and offers help to all personnel.

42. Is prompt when coming to work.

43. Conforms to hospital dress code.

44. Is rarely sick or absent from work due to health.

45. Stays available and accessible at all times when on duty.

46. Attends required inservice education programs, staff, and department meetings.

EMERGENCY DEPARTMENT NURSING ASSISTANT AND ORDERLY: PERFORMANCE EVALUATION

Name _____ Employment Date _____

Rating Period _____ To _____

Department _____ Job Title _____

Instructions: Using the following rating scale, indicate the quality of performance by placing the appropriate letter on the line to the left of the item.

U* – Unsatisfactory (does not meet job requirements)
S – Satisfactory (meets job requirements)
A – Above average (exceeds job requirements)
E* – Exceptional performance

RESPONSIBILITIES AND DUTIES

Patient Admission to Emergency Department:

_____ 1. Assists patient from car with wheelchair or stretcher to Emergency Department, then to stretcher in examination room.

_____

_____

_____ 2. Assists with obtaining information for patient and/or family for Emergency Department records.

_____

_____

_____ 3. Obtains vital signs as directed by RN:
   a. Blood pressure
   b. Heart rate (pulse)
   c. Respiration rate (describe—rapid, shallow, regular, deep, etc.)
   d. Temperature (orally, axillary, or rectally)

_____

_____

_____ 4. Documents on designated portions of outpatient record.

_____

_____

*The evaluator is expected to comment on all items rated "U" or "E."

_____ 5. Provides patient privacy.

_____

_____

_____ 6. Relates all patient/family questions to the RN.

_____

_____

Assists the RN as Instructed with:

_____ 7. Preparing patient for examination by physician

_____

_____

_____ 8. Cleaning patient in preparation for treatment

_____

_____

_____ 9. Draping and wrapping patient to maintain asepsis

_____

_____   _____

_____ 10. Connecting patient to heart monitor

_____

_____

_____ 11. Safety of patient:
a. Restraining as indicated
b. Ensures side rails are up when indicated
c. Assists patients in moving, sitting, and ambulating
d. Ensures patients are secured appropriately when transporting by wheelchair or stretcher.

_____

_____

_____ 12. Observing IV

_____

_____

_____ 13. Observing a patient receiving blood for signs and symptoms of reaction

_____

_____

_____ 14. Preop skin preparation

_____

_____

_____ 15. Application of casts by physician

_____

_____

_____ 16. Providing comfort measures

_____

_____

_____ 17. Intake and output

_____

_____

_____ 18. Oxygen therapy

_____

_____

_____ 19. Foley catheter (collecting specimens, securing bag, removing)

_____

_____

Assists RN in Caring for Patient with:

_____ 20. Central venous line

_____

_____

_____ 21. Chest tube

_____

_____

_____ 22. N.G. tube

_____

_____

_____ 23. Rotating tourniquets

_____

_____

_____ 24. Endotracheal tube/tracheostomy

_____

_____

_____ 25. Setting up sterile trays

_____

_____

_____ 26. Assists with specimen collection as requested:
   a. Urine—for U/A or clean catch
   b. Sputum
   c. Stool
   d. Other
   e. Labels all specimens with patient's name, date, time, and source
   f. Takes specimen to lab

   _____

   _____

_____ 27. Provides treatments as requested:
   a. Enema
   b. Insert rectal tube
   c. Give perineal care
   d. Test urine for sugar and acetone
   e. Apply hot or cold compresses
   f. Apply ice cap
   g. Apply ace bandages
   h. Give bedpan/urinal
   i. Provide fluids as instructed
   j. Weighing patient
   k. Applying vaginal pads

   _____

   _____

_____ 28. Assists RN in completing Emergency Department charge tickets.

   _____

   _____

_____ 29. Requisitions lab and X-ray work.

   _____

   _____

_____ 30. Assists RN in running errands, making calls, xeroxing, etc.

   _____

   _____

_____ 31. Supports patient during:
   a. Electrocardiogram
   b. Lab and X-ray procedures
   c. Treatments

   _____

   _____

_____ 32. Assists with admission of patient from Emergency Department to room:
   a. Takes patient to room; directs family to admitting as requested,
   b. Assists patient from stretcher or wheelchair to bed,
   c. Assists patient in moving personal belongings to room,
   d. Orients patient to surroundings, assuring patient is comfortable,
   e. Provides call light, bedside needs, and explains how to call nurse,
   f. Gives nurses on floor any pertinent information concerning patient.

_____ 33. Is familiar with Emergency Department and administration policies and procedures.

_____ 34. Is familiar with contents of trays, packs, and the location of equipment and supplies.

_____ 35. Assists in patient discharge from Emergency Department:
   a. Assists patient with clothing and collecting personal belongings,
   b. Assists patient to car,
   c. Ensures that all forms and requisitions are completed before patient discharge,
   d. Cleans stretchers and properly disposes of used supplies and equipment.

_____ 36. Is familiar with:
   a. All emergency equipment (Life Packs, MAST trousers, etc.),
   b. Care of orthopedic equipment,
   c. Care of CSR equipment and taking contaminated equipment back to CSR,
   d. Checks equipment for safety, proper operation, and tagging by maintenance.

_____ 37. Assists in maintaining ER supplies (checks supplies and reorders as indicated).

_____ 38. Maintains confidentiality of patient information.

_____ 39. Demonstrates practice of infection control principles:
    a. Handwashing
    b. Aseptic technique
    c. Sterile technique
    d. Adheres to isolation procedure

_____ 40. Acts rapidly and calmly during emergencies and provides the necessary materials called for by the RN.

_____ 41. Cooperates and offers help to all personnel.

_____ 42. Is prompt when coming to work.

_____ 43. Conforms to hospital dress code.

_____ 44. Is rarely sick or absent from work due to health.

_____ 45. Stays available and accessible at all times when on duty.

_____ 46. Attends required inservice education programs, staff, and department meetings.

EMERGENCY DEPARTMENT NURSING ASSISTANT AND ORDERLY: SCORING PROCEDURE

Instructions: Total the number of each item and multiply times the appropriate number. Add these totals to make the score.

U _____ × 0 = _____

S _____ × 1 = _____

A _____ × 2 = _____

E _____ × 3 = _____   _____ Total Score

Compare total score to the following scale to determine rank:

U	S	A	E
0 to 40	41 to 73	74 to 109	110 to 138

Overall Performance Review Score _____.

ALL ITEMS IN THE FOLLOWING SECTION MUST BE COMPLETED:

A. Interviewer's comments on overall review _____
_____
_____

B. Additional suggestions for overall work improvement and goals for next evaluation _____
_____
_____
_____

C. Self-objectives _____
_____
_____
_____

Date _____   Employee's signature

Date _____   Interviewer's signature

Date _____   Director of Nursing

MATERNAL AND CHILD HEALTH NURSING ASSISTANT: JOB DESCRIPTION

Position Requirements:
Good physical and mental health. Minimum of grammar school education, high school equivalent desirable. Genuine interest in welfare of the ill. Willingness to work under close supervision. Ability to follow written or verbal instructions effectively. Extended orientation including training for Maternal and Child Health Department.

Position Accountable For:
All nursing care behaviors described in the position description.

Position Accountable to:
Licensed Practical Nurse, Registered Nurse in charge of Department, Supervisor, Director of Nursing, patient, and family.

Position Summary:
Performs the functions of a Nursing Assistant in carrying out all assignments given by the Registered Nurse or Licensed Practical Nurse in the Department. Is accountable for all patient care she gives during a shift. Is responsible for adhering to all Standards of Nursing Care and for promoting teamwork among co-workers.

RESPONSIBILITIES AND DUTIES

1. Personal hygiene:
   a. Oral hygiene
   b. AM care (bathtub, shower, bed, etc.)
   c. PM care (back rub, etc.)
   d. Gives and removes bedpan
   e. Assists patients to and from bathroom
2. Provides clean linen when appropriate:
   a. makes unoccupied bed
   b. makes occupied bed
   c. makes postanesthetic bed
   d. changes and straightens linen to remove wrinkles
3. Positioning patients:
   a. Assists patient to find comfortable positions during labor,
   b. Positions patients correctly on delivery table (in stirrups, etc.),
   c. Changes patient's position appropriately and as frequently as instructed.

4. Dietary needs:
   a. Ensures the patient receives prescribed diet,
   b. Places tray conveniently for patient on overbed table with head of bed elevated,
   c. Assists or feeds patient as necessary,
   d. Encourages adequate food and fluid intake,
   e. Provides snacks at ordered time (especially for breast feeding mothers, diabetic patients, etc.),
   f. Removes tray and informs RN/LPN of patient's appetite (good, fair, poor, or refused).

5. Intake and Output:
   a. Posts I & O sheet and sign in room,
   b. Documents on I & O sheet all intake and output for the shift (including gomco, suction, Foley, etc.),
   c. Turns I & O sheet into RN/LPN 60 minutes prior to end of shift.

6. Specimen collection:
   Obtains specimens following RN/LPN instructions and labels all specimens with patient's full name, time, and initials.
   a. Urine
   b. Sputum
   c. Stool
   d. 24-hour urine
   e. Clean catch urine
   f. Lochia for C & S
   g. Takes specimens to lab and clocks time of lab slip.

7. Vital signs:
   Takes vital signs as instructed by RN/LPN:
   a. Temperature
   b. Heart rate (pulse)
   c. Respiration rate (including description)
   d. Blood pressure
   e. Notify RN/LPN of any change or abnormal finding.

8. Admissions:
   a. Escorts patient to room (patient room, labor room, delivery room as instructed) from Admitting or Emergency Department,
   b. Weighs patient,
   c. Assists patient to bed,
   d. Obtains vital signs and reports to RN/LPN,
   e. Ensures patient comfort and orients to surroundings,
   f. Assists RN/LPN with initial patient interview,
   g. Provides comfort kit.

9. Patient/family orientation:
   Instructs and explains the following:
   a. Call signal
   b. Thermostat
   c. Telephone
   d. TV

    e. Visitor policy
    f. Mealtimes
    g. Bathroom
    h. Introduce roommate
    i. Information booklet

10. Patient comfort:
    Responsible for providing:
    a. Patient privacy
    b. Skin care (keeps patient clean and dry)
    c. Limit of visitors when necessary
    d. Answers to call light promptly
    e. Additional comfort measures

11. Equipment and supplies:
    Familiar with the use and care of the following:
    a. CSR equipment (suction, gomco, K-pads, etc.)
    b. Ohio warming unit
    c. Delivery table
    d. Isolettes
    e. Infant resuscitation equipment
    f. Fetal heart monitor
    g. Duke inhaler
    h. Cleaning and wrapping of all instruments
    i. Location of all supplies needed
    j. Perineal light
    k. Linen packs

12. Safety:
    a. Keeps bed in low position and locked at all times,
    b. Ensures that patients are secured appropriately when transporting by wheelchair or stretcher,
    c. Assists patient in moving, sitting, or ambulating as necessary,
    d. Ensures that necessary articles are within easy reach (water, tissues, bedpan, telephone, etc.),
    e. Ensures that side rails remain in up position as indicated (past sedation, etc.),
    f. Ensures that smoking policy is enforced,
    g. Ensures that patient rooms remain free of clutter and all pathways are clear,
    h. Ensures that patient remains restrained as indicated.

13. Infection control:
    a. Uses good handwashing and aseptic technique,
    b. Uses sterile technique as indicated,
    c. Adheres to isolation procedure,
    d. Gives Foley catheter care to patients daily.

14. Assists the RN/LPN with the following:
    a. Observation of IVs
    b. Observation of patients receiving blood for signs and symptoms of reaction
    c. Foley catheter care
    d. N.G. tube

Within the scope of the job description assists with the following:

Prepartum Phase:
15. Times and notes character of contractions,
16. Assists physician or RN with vaginal exam,
17. Connects patient to Fetal Heart monitor,
18. Observes Fetal Heart monitor and reports to RN/LPN,
19. Encourages patient in proper breathing techniques,
20. Shaves and preps patient prior to delivery,
21. Finger prints patient for Newborn Identification Form.

Delivery:
22. Setting up for the delivery (sterile trays, etc.),
23. Assists the physician and RN/LPN as requested,
24. Assists the physician in resuscitation of the newborn,
25. Prepares Ohio warmer for newborn,
26. Completes newborn identification sheets, forms, and bracelets, places on both mother and newborn,
27. Orders and restocks supplies in delivery room.

Postpartum Phase:
28. Cleans patient following delivery,
29. Transports patient to room,
30. Transports newborn to nursery,
31. Checks and massages fundus,
32. Checks lochia (for amount, color, and consistency),
33. Assists RN in teaching patient concerning self-care and care of the newborn,
34. Cleans suture sites as instructed; changes dressings as instructed.

Within the scope of the job description provides the following care for the newborn:
35. Bathing
36. Weighing, measuring chest and head daily
37. Cord care daily
38. Application of $AGNO_3$ drops to eyes
39. Suction (bulb syringe)
40. Monitor of 0_2 therapy
41. Bilirubin light and mask
42. Application of U-Bag for urine specimen
43. Feeding of infants (bottle feeding for normal newborn as well as premature or cleft lip and/or palate), reports amount and how tolerated to RN/LPN
44. Vital signs

45. Observation of respiratory status
    a. flaring of nostrils
    b. retracting
    c. cyanosis
    d. grunting
46. Circumcision care
47. Assists with holding infant for the following procedures:
    a. spinal tap
    b. femoral sticks
    c. circumcisions
    d. bladder taps

Prior to discharge of the patient and newborn assists with the following:

48. Reinforces patient home care instructions (Distributes Gift Packs and Pamphlets),
49. Checks patient and newborn's identification bands for compliance,
50. Checks newborn Identification form with patient to ensure identical numbers—has patient sign,
51. Collects patient's personal items,
52. Escorts patient and newborn to car by wheelchair.

General evaluation items:

53. Supports and adheres to nursing service and administrative policies and procedures,
54. Cooperates and offers help to other nursing service departments as requested,
55. Relates all patient questions to RN/LPN,
56. Conforms to department dress code,
57. Is rarely sick or absent from work due to health,
58. Is prompt and attends report,
59. Is available and accessible at all times when on duty,
60. Attends inservice education programs, staff, and unit meetings.

MATERNAL AND CHILD HEALTH NURSING ASSISTANT: PERFORMANCE EVALUATION

Name _____ Employment Date _____

Rating Period _____ To _____

Department _____ Job Title _____

Instructions: Using the following rating scale, indicate the quality of performance by placing the appropriate letter on the line to the left of the item.

U* – Unsatisfactory (does not meet job requirements)
S – Satisfactory (meets job requirements)
A – Above average (exceeds job requirements)
E* – Exceptional performance

RESPONSIBILITIES AND DUTIES

_____ 1. Personal hygiene:
     a. Oral hygiene
     b. AM care (bath-tub, shower, bed, etc.)
     c. PM care (back rub, etc.)
     d. Gives and removes bedpan
     e. Assists patients to and from bathroom

_____

_____

_____ 2. Provides clean linen when appropriate:
     a. Makes unoccupied bed
     b. Makes occupied bed
     c. Makes postanesthetic bed
     d. Changes and straightens linen to remove wrinkles

_____

_____

_____ 3. Positioning patients:
     a. Assists patient to find comfortable positions during labor,
     b. Positions patients correctly on delivery table (in stirrups, etc.),
     c. Changes patient's position appropriately and as frequently as instructed.

_____

_____

*The evaluator is expected to comment on all items rated "U" or "E."

_____ 4. Dietary needs:
   a. Ensures the patient receives prescribed diet,
   b. Places tray conveniently for patient on overbed table with head of bed elevated,
   c. Assists or feeds patient as necessary,
   d. Encourages adequate food and fluid intake,
   e. Provides snacks at ordered time (especially for breast feeding mothers, diabetic patients, etc.),
   f. Removes tray and informs RN/LPN of patient's appetite (good, fair, poor, or refused).

_____ 5. Intake and output:
   a. Posts I & O sheet and sign in room,
   b. Documents on I & O sheet all intake and output for the shift (including gomco, suction, Foley, etc.),
   c. Turns I & O sheet into RN/LPN 60 minutes prior to end of shift.

_____ 6. Specimen collection:
   Obtains specimens following RN/LPN instructions and labels all specimens with patient's full name, time, and initials.
   a. Urine
   b. Sputum
   c. Stool
   d. 24-hour urine
   e. Clean catch urine
   f. Lochia for C & S
   g. Takes specimens to lab and clocks time on lab slip.

_____ 7. Vital signs: Takes vital signs as instructed by RN/LPN:
   a. Temperature
   b. Heart rate (pulse)
   c. Respiration rate (including description)
   d. Blood pressure
   e. Notify RN/LPN of any change or abnormal finding.

_____ 8. Admissions:
   a. Escorts patient to room (patient room, labor room, delivery room as instructed) from Admitting or Emergency Department,

       b. Weighs patient,

       c. Assists patient to bed,

       d. Obtains vital signs and reports to RN/LPN,

       e. Ensures patient comfort and orients to surroundings,

       f. Assists RN/LPN with initial patient interview,

       g. Provides comfort kit.

_____

_____

_____ 9. Patient and family orientation: Instructs and explains the following:

       a. Call signal

       b. Thermostat

       c. Telephone

       d. T.V.

       e. Visitor policy

       f. Meal times

       g. Bathroom

       h. Introduce roommate

       i. Information booklet

_____ 10. Patient comfort: Responsible for providing:

       a. Patient privacy

       b. Skin care (keeps patient clean and dry)

       c. Limit visitors when necessary

       d. Answers call light promptly

       e. Additional comfort measures

_____

_____

_____ 11. Equipment and supplies: Familiar with the use and care of the following:

       a. CSR equipment (suction, gomco, K-pads, etc.)

       b. Ohio warming unit

       c. Delivery table

       d. Isolettes

       e. Infant resuscitation equipment

       f. Fetal heart monitor

       g. Duke inhaler

       h. Cleaning and wrapping of all instruments

       i. Location of all supplies needed

       j. Perineal light

       k. Linen packs

_____

_____

_____ 12. Safety:
    a. Keeps bed in low position and locked at all times,
    b. Ensures that patients are secured appropriately when transporting by wheelchair or stretcher,
    c. Assists patient in moving, sitting, or ambulating as necessary,
    d. Ensures that necessary articles are within easy reach (water, tissues, bedpan, telephone, etc.),
    e. Ensures that side rails remain in up position as indicated (past sedation, etc.),
    f. Ensures that smoking policy is enforced,
    g. Ensures that patient rooms remain free of clutter and all pathways are clear,
    h. Ensures that patient remains restrained as indicated.

_____

_____

_____ 13. Infection control:
    a. Uses good handwashing and aseptic technique,
    b. Uses sterile technique as indicated,
    c. Adheres to isolation procedure,
    d. Gives Foley catheter care to patients daily.

_____

_____

_____ 14. Assists the RN/LPN with the following:
    a. Observation of IVs
    b. Observation of patients receiving blood for signs and symptoms of reaction
    c. Foley catheter care
    d. N.G. tube

_____

_____

Within the scope of the job description, assists with the following:

Prepartum phase:

_____ 15. Times and notes character of contractions.

_____

_____

_____ 16. Assists physician or RN with vaginal exam.

_____

_____

_____ 17. Connects patient to fetal heart monitor.

_____

_____

_____ 18. Observes fetal heart monitor and reports to RN/LPN.

_____

_____

_____ 19. Encourages patient in proper breathing techniques.

_____

_____

_____ 20. Shaves and preps patient prior to delivery.

_____

_____

_____ 21. Fingerprints patient for newborn identification form.

_____

_____

Delivery:

_____ 22. Setting up for the delivery (sterile trays, etc.).

_____

_____

_____ 23. Assists the physician and RN/LPN as requested.

_____

_____

_____ 24. Assists the physician in resuscitation of the newborn.

_____

_____

_____ 25. Prepares Ohio warmer for newborn.

_____

_____

_____ 26. Completes newborn identification sheets, forms, and bracelets, places on both mother and newborn.

_____

_____

_____ 27. Orders and restocks supplies in delivery room.

_____

_____

Postpartum phase:

_____ 28. Cleans patient following delivery.

_____ 29. Transports patient to room.

_____ 30. Transports newborn to nursery.

_____ 31. Checks and massages fundus.

_____ 32. Checks lochia (for amount, color, and consistency).

_____ 33. Assists RN in teaching patient concerning self-care and care of the newborn.

_____ 34. Cleans suture sites as instructed; changes dressings as instructed.

Within the scope of the job description, provides the following care for the newborn:

_____ 35. Bathing.

_____ 36. Weighing, measuring chest and head daily.

_____ 37. Cord care daily.

_____ 38. Application of AGNO3 drops to eyes.

_____

_____

_____ 39. Suction (bulb syringe).

_____

_____

_____ 40. Monitor of O_2 therapy.

_____

_____

_____ 41. Bilirubin light and mask.

_____

_____

_____ 42. Application of U-Bag for urine specimen.

_____

_____

_____ 43. Feeding of infants (bottle feeding for normal newborn as well as premature or cleft lip and/or palate), reports amount and how tolerated to RN/LPN.

_____

_____

_____ 44. Vital signs.

_____

_____

_____ 45. Observation of respiratory status:
   a. Flaring of nostrils
   b. Retracting
   c. Cyanosis
   d. Grunting

_____

_____

_____ 46. Circumcision care.

_____

_____

_____ 47. Assists with holding infant for the following procedures:
   a. Spinal tap
   b. Femoral sticks

    c. Circumcisions

    d. Bladder taps

_____

_____

Prior to discharge of the patient and newborn:

_____ 48. Reinforces patient home care instructions (distributes gift packs and pamphlets).

_____

_____

_____ 49. Checks patient's and newborn's identification bands for compliance.

_____

_____

_____ 50. Checks newborn identification form with patient to ensure identical numbers; has patient sign.

_____

_____

_____ 51. Collects patient's personal items.

_____

_____

_____ 52. Escorts patient and newborn to car by wheelchair.

_____

_____

General evaluation items:

_____ 53. Supports and adheres to nursing service and administrative policies and procedures.

_____

_____

_____ 54. Cooperates and offers help to other nursing service departments as requested.

_____

_____

_____ 55. Relates all patient questions to RN/LPN.

_____

_____

_____ 56. Conforms to department dress code.

_____ 57. Is rarely sick or absent from work due to health.

_____ 58. Is prompt and attends report.

_____ 59. Is available and accessible at all times when on duty.

_____ 60. Attends inservice education programs, staff, and unit meetings.

MATERNAL AND CHILD HEALTH NURSING ASSISTANT: SCORING PROCEDURE

Instructions: Total the number of each item and multiply times the appropriate number. Add these totals to make the score.

U _____ × 0 = _____

S _____ × 1 = _____

A _____ × 2 = _____

E _____ × 3 = _____   _____ Total Score

Compare total score to the following scale to determine rank:

U	S	A	E
0 to 53	54 to 95	96 to 143	144 to 180

Overall Performance Review Score _____.

ALL ITEMS IN THE FOLLOWING SECTION MUST BE COMPLETED:

A. Interviewer's comments on overall review _____

_____

_____

B. Additional suggestions for overall work improvement and goals for next evaluation _____

_____

_____

C. Self-objectives _____

_____

_____

_____

_____   _____
Date   Employee's signature

_____   _____
Date   Interviewer's signature

_____   _____
Date   Director of Nursing

SURGICAL TECHNICIAN: JOB DESCRIPTION

Position Requirements: Good physical and mental health. High School education preferred. Genuine interest in Surgical Nursing. Willingness to work under supervision. Ability to follow written or verbal instructions. Prior training as a technician in Surgical Nursing preferred.

Position Accountable for: All nursing care described in position description.

Position Accountable to: Licensed Practical Nurse, Registered Nurse in charge, Supervisor, and Director of Nursing, patient, and family

Position Summary: Within the Surgical Department, the technician shall assist in nursing care and surgical services under the Registered Nurses' supervision and according to job description and hospital policies.

RESPONSIBILITIES AND DUTIES

Performs delegated duties as a member of the nursing team:
1. Assists in preparing the preoperative site.
2. Under the Registered Nurse's supervision, assists with nursing activities required during the operation (i.e., handling of instruments, sponges, sutures, catheter, and drains).
3. Assists in keeping operating room clean at all times.

When transporting patient to Operating Room, assists the nurse in:
4. Checking the chart for complete preoperative check list and all required records and reports.
5. Confirming correctness of surgical site.
6. Securing safe transport of patient from bed to operating room.

Specific scrub duties:
7. Assists circulating nurse in setting up room with instruments and supplies for the case scheduled in that room. Checks doctor's reference cards for special needs of the surgeon doing the case.
8. Assists in properly positioning patient on table.
9. Scrubbing, gowning, and gloving procedure:
   a. Follows steps of scrubbing procedure according to established policy,
   b. Properly dons sterile gown and gloves.

Preparation of sterile setup:

10. Arranges instruments on Mayo according to routine for given procedure.
11. Obtains instruments from autoclave and transports them to sterile field without contamination.
12. Counts all sponges with circulating nurse.
13. Gowns and gloves other scrubbed personnel.
14. Assists in draping procedure.
    a. Folds towels and hands to surgeon correctly,
    b. Avoids reaching over nonsterile table,
    c. Stands well back from nonsterile table when unfolding sterile sheets over patient,
    d. Keeps hands at table level,
    e. Attaches suction tubing and cautery cord to drapes,
    f. Attaches light handles, if used.
15. Identifies, prepares, and correctly passes instruments to the surgeon.
16. Keeps operative field neat, clean, and dry.
17. Asks quietly for additional supplies and limits conversation to a minimum.

Practices good aseptic technique:

18. Recognizes and verbalizes breaks in technique by self and others.
19. Within sterile field.
    a. Limits traffic,
    b. Controls own movements within sterile field,
    c. Turns back to nonsterile objects in room when passing them.
20. Keeps hands at waist level.
21. Is familiar with and adheres to surgical department policies and procedures.
22. Confirms correctness of sponge count when giving the suture for closing the peritoneum in abdominal operations.
23. Has final dressings ready when first layer of wound has been closed.
24. Maintains sterile setup until patient has left room. Assists with cleanup of surgical suite:
    a. Places disposables in receptacle, isolates needles, blades, and sharp objects to prevent injury to others,
    b. Opens used instruments, places in water, and washes with instrument detergent. Separates soiled instruments into basin. Keeps delicate instruments separate,
    c. Properly disposes of linen, trash, sponges, etc.,
    d. Restocks extra supplies and unused equipment.
25. Conforms to dress code policy.
    a. Wears proper attire,
    b. Wears lab coat when not in operating room/recovery room,
    c. Keeps all facial and head hair completely covered,
    d. Changes masks between cases,
    e. Removes gown and gloves before leaving operating suite.
26. Helps to orient and instruct new personnel in functions, activities, and procedures.

27. Inspects department regularly for proper equipment functions.
28. Maintains adequate stock of equipment and supplies.
29. Promotes good harmonious relationships and favorable attitudes among the health care team.
30. Attends required inservice education programs.
31. Evaluates surgical technician orientation policies and procedures when requested and recommends revisions as necessary.
32. Attends department and staff meetings.
33. Is rarely sick or absent from work.
34. Stays available and accessible at all times when on duty and when on call.

SURGICAL TECHNICIAN: PERFORMANCE EVALUATION

Name _____ Employment Date _____

Rating Period _____ To _____

Department _____ Job Title _____

Instructions: Using the following rating scale, indicate the quality of performance by placing the appropriate letter on the line to the left of the item.

U* – Unsatisfactory (does not meet job requirements)
S – Satisfactory (meets job requirements)
A – Above average (exceeds job requirements)
E* – Exceptional performance

RESPONSIBILITIES AND DUTIES

Performs delegated duties as a member of the nursing team:

_____ 1. Assists in preparing the preoperative site.

_____

_____

_____ 2. Under the Registered Nurse's supervision, assists with nursing activities required during the operation (i.e., handling of instruments, sponges, sutures, catheter, and drains).

_____

_____

_____ 3. Assists in keeping operating room clean at all times.

_____

_____

When transporting patient to Operating Room, assists the nurse in:

_____ 4. Checking the chart for complete preoperative checklist and all required records and reports.

_____

_____

_____

*The evaluator is expected to comment on all items rated "U" or "E."

_____ 5. Confirming correctness of surgical site.

_____

_____

_____ 6. Securing safe transport of patient from bed to operating room.

_____

_____

Specific scrub duties:

_____ 7. Assists circulating nurse in setting up room with instruments and supplies for the case scheduled in that room. Checks doctor's reference cards for special needs of the surgeon doing the case.

_____

_____

_____ 8. Assists in properly positioning patient on table.

_____

_____

_____ 9. Scrubbing, gowning, and gloving procedure:
   a. Follows steps of scrubbing procedure according to established policy,
   b. Properly dons sterile gown and gloves.

_____

_____

Preparation of sterile setup:

_____ 10. Arranges instruments on Mayo according to routine for given procedure.

_____

_____

_____ 11. Obtains instruments from autoclave and transports them to sterile field without contamination.

_____

_____

_____ 12. Counts all sponges with circulating nurse.

_____

_____

_____ 13. Gowns and gloves other scrubbed personnel.

_____

_____

_____ 14. Assists in draping procedure:
   a. Folds towels and hands to surgeon correctly,
   b. Avoids reaching over nonsterile table,
   c. Stands well back from nonsterile table when unfolding sterile sheets over patient,
   d. Keeps hands at table level,
   e. Attaches suction tubing and cautery cord to drapes,
   f. Attaches light handles, if used.

_____

_____

_____ 15. Identifies, prepares, and correctly passes instruments to the surgeon.

_____

_____

_____ 16. Keeps operative field neat, clean, and dry.

_____

_____

_____ 17. Asks quietly for additional supplies and limits conversation to a minimum.

_____

_____

Practices good aseptic technique:

_____ 18. Recognizes and verbalizes breaks in technique by self and others.

_____

_____

_____ 19. Within sterile field:
   a. Limits traffic,
   b. Controls own movements within sterile field,
   c. Turns back to nonsterile objects in room when passing them.

_____ 20. Keeps hands at waist level.

_____

_____

_____ 21. Is familiar with and adheres to surgical department policies and procedures.

_____

_____

_____ 22. Confirms correctness of sponge count when giving the suture for closing the peritoneum in abdominal operations.

_____ 23. Has final dressings ready when first layer of wound has been closed.

_____ 24. Maintains sterile setup until patient has left room. Assists with cleanup of surgical suite:
   a. Places disposables in receptacle, isolates needles, blades, and sharp objects to prevent injury to others,
   b. Opens used instruments, places in water, and washes with instrument detergent. Separates soiled instruments into basin. Keeps delicate instruments separate,
   c. Properly disposes of linen, trash, sponges, etc.,
   d. Restocks extra supplies and unused equipment.

_____ 25. Conforms to dress code policy:
   a. Wears proper attire,
   b. Wears lab coat when not in operating room/recovery room,
   c. Keeps all facial and head hair completely covered,
   d. Changes masks between cases,
   e. Removes gown and gloves before leaving operating suite.

_____ 26. Helps to orient and instruct new personnel in functions, activities, and procedures.

_____ 27. Inspects department regularly for proper equipment functions.

_____ 28. Maintains adequate stock of equipment and supplies.

_____ 29. Promotes good harmonious relationships and favorable attitudes among the health care team.

_____

_____

_____ 30. Attends required inservice education programs.

_____

_____

_____ 31. Evaluates surgical technician orientation policies and procedures when requested and recommends revisions as necessary.

_____

_____

_____ 32. Attends department and staff meetings.

_____

_____

_____ 33. Is rarely sick or absent from work.

_____

_____

_____ 34. Stays available and accessible at all times when on duty and when on call.

_____

_____

SURGICAL TECHNICIAN: SCORING PROCEDURE

Instructions: Total the number of each item and multiply times the appropriate number. Add these totals to make the score.

U _____ $\times 0 =$ _____

S _____ $\times 1 =$ _____

A _____ $\times 2 =$ _____

E _____ $\times 3 =$ _____   _____ Total Score

Compare total score to the following scale to determine rank:

U	S	A	E
0 to 30	31 to 53	54 to 81	82 to 102

Overall Performance Review Score _____.

ALL ITEMS IN THE FOLLOWING SECTION MUST BE COMPLETED:

A. Interviewer's comments on overall review _____

_____

_____

B. Additional suggestions for overall work improvement and goals for next evaluation _____

_____

_____

C. Self-objectives _____

_____

_____

_____

_____   _____

Date   Employee's signature

_____   _____

Date   Interviewer's signature

_____   _____

Date   Director of Nursing

CENTRAL SERVICE TECHNICIAN: JOB DESCRIPTION

Position Requirements:	Good physical and mental health. High School education or equivalent. Ability to follow written or verbal instructions effectively. Willing to accept responsibility. Must be neat and well groomed.
Position Accountable to:	Director of Nursing, Central Service Department Supervisor, patient, and family.
Position Accountable for:	All behaviors described in position description.
Position Summary:	Performs duties involving the care, packaging, cleaning, and charging of items and supplies utilized in the hospital.

The Central Service Technician will perform the following duties:

1. Will be familiar with all Central Service policies and procedures.
2. Is familiar with all Infection Control policies and procedures specific to his/her area.
3. Perform ATTEST weekly.
4. Autoclave:
   a. Check autoclave at the beginning of his/her shift,
   b. Begin new chart with each new load,
   c. Clean instruments prior to wrapping,
   d. Double wrap instruments properly,
   e. Log each load in log book with date, time, pressure, temperature, contents, and signature,
   f. Place blue and white sticker with date autoclaved and expiration marked,
   g. Check expiration dates of all sterile equipment and trays,
   h. Check Sterile trays and equipment for: contamination, tears, holes, and moisture,
   i. Autoclave all outdated or contaminated equipment and return to appropriate department.
5. Pick up charge slips on each unit daily.
6. Log all charges as indicated.

Machines—Suction, Gomco, and K-Pads:

7. Clean after each use,
8. Replace tubing after each use,
9. Place orange sticker showing date cleaned and initials on each machine,
10. Ensure that equipment has been checked for safety and proper functioning.

Isolation carts:
   a. Stock cart according to type Isolation ordered.
   b. Charge daily for cart.
   c. Check cart twice during shift for needed supplies.
   d. Empty and clean cart when Isolation is discontinued.
11. Restock IV trays.
12. Restock Treatment Rooms.
13. Inventory Supplies, order, and stock as needed.
14. Return to Central Supply when a Code 9 is called.
15. Update Central Service Listing Book as needed and stock supplies accordingly.
16. Attend required inservice programs and staff meetings.
17. Cooperate and offer help to all personnel.
18. Conform to hospital dress code.
19. Support nursing service and administration policies and procedures.
20. Is rarely sick or absent from work due to health.
21. Is prompt.
22. Stay available and accessible at all times while on duty.

CENTRAL SERVICE TECHNICIAN: PERFORMANCE EVALUATION

Name _____ Employment Date _____

Rating Period _____ To _____

Department _____ Job Title _____

Instructions: Using the following rating scale, indicate the quality of performance by placing the appropriate letter on the line to the left of the item.

U* – Unsatisfactory (does not meet job requirements)
S – Satisfactory (meets job requirements)
A – Above average (exceeds job requirements)
E* – Exceptional performance

The Central Service Technician will perform the following duties:

_____ 1. Will be familiar with all Central Service policies and procedures.

_____

_____

_____ 2. Is familiar with all Infection Control policies and procedures specific to his/her area.

_____

_____

_____ 3. Perform ATTEST weekly.

_____

_____

_____ 4. Autoclave:
   a. Check autoclave at the beginning of his/her shift,
   b. Begin new chart with each new load,
   c. Clean instruments prior to wrapping,
   d. Double wrap instruments properly,
   e. Log each load in logbook with date, time, pressure, temperature, contents, and signature,
   f. Place blue and white sticker with date autoclaved and expiration marked,
   g. Check expiration dates of all sterile equipment and trays,
   h. Check sterile trays and equipment for: contamination, tears, holes, and moisture,

---

*The evaluator is expected to comment on all items rated "U" or "E."

      i. Autoclave all outdated or contaminated equipment and return to appropriate department.

———— 5. Pick up charge slips on each unit daily.

———— 6. Log all charges as indicated.

Machines—Suction, Gomco, and K-Pads:

———— 7. Clean after each use.

———— 8. Replace tubing after each use.

———— 9. Place orange sticker showing date cleaned and initials on each machine.

———— 10. Ensure that equipment has been checked for safety and proper functioning.

Isolation carts:

———— a. Stock cart according to type isolation ordered.

———— b. Charge daily for cart.

———— c. Check cart twice during shift for needed supplies.

_____ d.   Empty and clean cart when isolation is discontinued.

_____ 11.   Restock IV trays.

_____ 12.   Restock treatment rooms.

_____ 13.   Inventory supplies, order and stock as needed.

_____ 14.   Return to Central Supply when a Code 9 is called.

_____ 15.   Update Central Service listing book as needed and stock supplies accordingly.

_____ 16.   Attend required inservice programs and staff meetings.

_____ 17.   Cooperate and offer help to all personnel.

_____ 18.   Conform to hospital dress code.

_____ 19.   Support nursing service and administration policies and procedures.

_____ 20.   Is rarely sick or absent from work due to health.

_____ 21. Is prompt.

_____

_____

_____ 22. Stay available and accessible at all times while on duty.

_____

_____

CENTRAL SERVICE TECHNICIAN: SCORING PROCEDURE

Instructions: Total the number of each item and multiply times the appropriate number. Add these totals to make the score.

U _____ × 0 = _____

S _____ × 1 = _____

A _____ × 2 = _____

E _____ × 3 = _____   _____ Total Score

Compare total score to the following scale to determine rank:

U	S	A	E
0 to 22	23 to 41	42 to 61	62 to 78

Overall Performance Review Score _____.

ALL ITEMS IN THE FOLLOWING SECTION MUST BE COMPLETED:

A. Interviewer's comments on overall review _____
_____
_____

B. Additional suggestions for overall work improvement and goals for next evaluation _____
_____
_____

C. Self-objectives _____
_____
_____
_____

_____
Date

_____
Date

_____
Date

Employee's signature

Interviewer's signature

Director of Nursing

UNIT SECRETARY: JOB DESCRIPTION

Position Requirements:
Good physical and mental health. High School Graduate, Unit Secretary training or experience preferred. Must be neat, well groomed, and have a pleasing personality and voice. Must be willing to accept responsibility and instructions.

Position Accountable to:
Licensed Practical Nurse, Registered Nurse, Head Nurse, Supervisor, Director of Nursing, and patient and family.

Position Accountable for:
All behaviors described in the position description.

Position Summary:
The Unit Secretary, under the direction and supervision of the charge nurse of the unit, is responsible for manning the nursing station and performing clerical and receptionist duties, and requisitioning supplies, equipment, and services from other departments. The unit secretary should be emotionally stable and mature, accurate and organized, and flexible in her dealings with other people.

RESPONSIBILITIES AND DUTIES

1. Conforms to hospital dress code.
2. Supports and adheres to hospital and nursing service policies and procedures.
3. Is rarely sick or absent from work due to health.
4. Is prompt.
5. Meets with charge nurse concerning daily assignments and work related problems and needs.
6. Maintains good employee relations, interdepartmental and public relations.
7. Attends inservice education programs.
8. Keeps up-to-date in unit activities.
9. Assumes responsibility for establishing and maintaining a satisfactory physical environment in the nursing station.
10. Acts as receptionist for the nursing station, answering inquiries of a general nature by: patients, visitors, other departments, nursing staff, and physicians, assisting them in a friendly and cooperative manner:
    a. Takes and relays messages to personnel on the unit,
    b. Assists volunteers or delivers gifts, flowers, and mail to patients on the unit,
    c. Runs errands when necessary for nursing staff.

11. Activates paging system for routine calls, Code 9, and other emergencies as directed.

12. Coordinates and provides routine services, supplies, and equipment to the nursing unit:
    a. Requisitions supplies, equipment and maintenance and repair services, as directed, and prepares related forms,
    b. Prepares diet and juice lists and sends them to dietary department. Calls in diet orders,
    c. Requests hospital services such as chaplain, television, and social service for patients by placing calls to appropriate areas.

13. Prepares requisitions for diagnostic and therapeutic services for patients and coordinates appointments with other departments:
    a. Accepts and schedules appointments, makes appropriate entries in the Kardex, completes required hospital forms, and notifies appropriate staff and patients,
    b. Routes charts to departments as required for diagnostic and treatment procedures or consultation.

14. Performs clerical duties related to procedures such as admission, discharge, transfer, death:
    a. Notifies the appropriate departments and staff of patient disposition,
    b. Assembles and prepares the appropriate charts and forms,
    c. Ensures patient valuables and personal items are properly handled and accounted for,
    d. Updates patient census and disposition of records and reports,
    e. Routes patient records according to established procedures.

15. Keeps patient's records current in specific areas:
    a. Prepares physicians' order for checking by professional nurse, following transcription procedure,
    b. Charts routine TPR, BP, and other information,
    c. Records intake and output on patient's chart and enters required information on diabetic flow records,
    d. Files reports of tests, procedures, and consultation,
    e. Copies and computes other data as directed,
    f. Keeps charts in order with all forms properly identified.

16. Keeps medical record file in proper order and pulls charts as needed and sees that only authorized persons have access to patient records.

17. Keeps stock and equipment inventories.

18. Manages interdepartmental and patients' mail.

19. Assists with or maintains hospital and unit records (i.e., NPO lists, time sheets, census report, master assignment sheet, call-in book).

20. Transmits reports as directed.

21. Maintains unit library in order and keeps records of material on loan.

22. Performs other duties as directed by supervisor.

23. Maintains contact with departments furnishing supplies and equipment and services to the unit.

24. Uses established hospital and nursing hierarchial structure for problems and grievances.

UNIT SECRETARY: PERFORMANCE EVALUATION

Name _____ Employment date _____

Rating Period _____ To _____

Department _____ Job Title _____

Instructions: Using the following rating scale, indicate the quality of performance by placing the appropriate letter on the line to the left of the item.

U* – Unsatisfactory (does not meet job requirements)
S – Satisfactory (meets job requirements)
A – Above average (exceeds job requirements)
E* – Exceptional performance

RESPONSIBILITIES AND DUTIES

_____ 1. Conforms to hospital dress code.

_____

_____

_____ 2. Supports and adheres to hospital and nursing service policies and procedures.

_____

_____

_____ 3. Is rarely sick or absent from work due to health.

_____

_____

_____ 4. Is prompt.

_____

_____

_____ 5. Meets with charge nurse concerning daily assignments and work related problems and needs.

_____

_____

*The evaluator is expected to comment on all items rated "U" or "E."

_____ 6. Maintains good employee relations, interdepartmental, and public relations.

_____

_____

_____ 7. Attends inservice education programs.

_____

_____

_____ 8. Keeps up-to-date in unit activities.

_____

_____

_____ 9. Assumes responsibility for establishing and maintaining a satisfactory physical environment in the nursing station.

_____

_____

_____ 10. Acts as receptionist for the nursing station, answering inquiries of a general nature by patients, visitors, other departments, nursing staff, and physicians, assisting them in a friendly and cooperative manner.
   a. Takes and relays messages to personnel on the unit,
   b. Assists volunteers or delivers gifts, flowers, and mail to patients on the unit,
   c. Runs errands when necessary for nursing staff.

_____

_____

_____ 11. Activates paging system for routine calls, Code 9, and other emergencies as directed.

_____ 12. Coordinates and provides routine services, supplies, and equipment to the nursing unit:
   a. Requisitions supplies, equipment and maintenance and repair services as directed and prepares related forms,
   b. Prepares diet and juice lists and sends them to dietary department. Calls in diet orders,
   c. Requests hospital services, such as chaplain, television, and social service for patients by placing calls to appropriate areas.

_____

_____

_____ 13. Prepares requisitions for diagnostic and therapeutic services for patients and coordinates appointments with other departments:
a. Accepts and schedules appointments, makes appropriate entries in the Kardex, completes required hospital forms, and notifies appropriate staff and the patients.
b. Routes charts to departments as required for diagnostic and treatment procedures or consultation.

_____

_____

_____ 14. Performs clerical duties related to procedures such as admission, discharge, transfer, death:
a. Notifies the appropriate departments and staff of patient disposition,
b. Assembles and prepares the appropriate charts and forms,
c. Ensures patient valuables and personal items are properly handled and accounted for,
d. Updates patient census and disposition records and reports,
e. Routes patient records according to established procedures.

_____

_____

_____ 15. Keeps patients' records current in specific areas such as:
a. Prepares physician's order for checking by professional nurse, following transcription procedure,
b. Charts routine TPR, BP, and other information,
c. Records intake and output on patient's chart and enters required information on diabetic flow records,
d. Files reports of tests, procedures, and consultation,
e. Copies and computes other data as directed,
f. Keeps charts in order with all forms properly identified.

_____

_____

_____ 16. Keeps medical record file in proper order and pulls charts as needed and sees that only authorized persons have access to patient records.

_____

_____

_____ 17. Keeps stock and equipment inventories.

_____

_____

_____ 18. Manages interdepartmental and patients' mail.

_____

_____

_____ 19. Assists with or maintains hospital and unit records (i.e., NPO lists, time sheets, census report, master assignment sheet, call-in book).

_____

_____

_____ 20. Transmits reports as directed.

_____

_____

_____ 21. Maintains unit library in order and keeps records of material on loan.

_____

_____

_____ 22. Performs other duties as directed by supervisor.

_____

_____

_____ 23. Maintains contact with departments furnishing supplies and equipment and services to the unit.

_____

_____

_____ 24. Uses established hospital and nursing hierarchial structure for problems and grievances.

_____

_____

UNIT SECRETARY: SCORING PROCEDURE

Instructions: Total the number of each item and multiply times the appropriate number. Add these totals to make the score.

U _____ × 0 = _____

S _____ × 1 = _____

A _____ × 2 = _____

E _____ × 3 = _____   _____ Total Score

Compare total score to the following scale to determine rank:

U	S	A	E
0 to 21	22 to 37	38 to 57	58 to 72

Overall Performance Review Score _____ .

ALL ITEMS IN THE FOLLOWING SECTION MUST BE COMPLETED:

A. Interviewer's comments on overall review _____
_____
_____

B. Additional suggestions for overall work improvement and goals for next evaluation _____
_____
_____

C. Self-objectives _____
_____
_____
_____

_____   _____
Date   Employee's signature

_____   _____
Date   Interviewer's signature

_____   _____
Date   Director of Nursing

Index